Barbell

Training

Step-to-step Guide to Get Fit and Move Pain Free

(A Weight Training Guide for Strength & Fitness That Won't Go Out of Fashion)

Torrey Frami

Published By **Elena Holly**

Torrey Frami

Barbell Training: Step-to-step Guide to Get Fit and Move Pain Free (A Weight Training Guide for Strength & Fitness That Won't Go Out of Fashion)

ISBN   978-1-77485-981-0

Legal & Disclaimer

Table of contents

Chapter 1: Tactical Barbell Overview

Tactical Bar-Bell can be used to strengthen and condition athletes in many different fitness domains. TB1 insured strength. This publication is about conditioning. Researchers have unique strength and condition requirements, according to your definition of an operational athlete. An infantry soldier who is eliminated from an operation will not work in the exact same way as a SWAT agent. Bobby professional worker might not teach in the exact same way as Johnny SWAT. They simply want to be exceptionally strong and ready for any given task. Johnny SWAT will require an increased level of aerobic/endurance conditioning for the infantry soldier. The benefits of aerobic training are not limited to office workers. They may need to do it for just 30 seconds. The aims of office workers can vary. However, they may also change along with your interests or way of living. Next year, which division worker wants to conduct an adventure race? Maybe the infantry soldiers chooses BJJ. The training required to alter. You may want to switch to energy systems or focus on potency. TBI and TBI Two give you the ability to move within those training parameters. You will have the ability to move your practice around if your interests shift towards experience racing. Continued focus on maximising maximum potency for three more weeks. This will help you to fix your conditioning. If you want to be a high-performance, highly-motivated working athlete, this application is for you. This novel will show you how to enhance your time strategies, increase workout capacity and muscle endurance, as well as boost volatile energy. In this book, you'll also be taught how to integrate all of these with your existing intensity training. What is the secret to becoming a master at everything? These are the essential things you should do to be able to take your journey from being a host to owning a 600lb weight loss and running a 5km race in just 9 minutes. Two essential skills are required: understanding how to PRIORITIZE as well as the ways you can be EFFICIENT. It is essential to learn how to coach each of the systems in the most productive way. Performance is important because runners can't afford not to train in the best possible way. There are many skills you need to master. Your time and energy are likely to be scarce and limited. Instead of spending time trying to build your heart using eight different exercises while foam rolling and working with a medicine balls, you'll need to focus on less, more direct moves. There are many options, such as boards, hanging leg raises, ab rollers, dead lifts or squats. It is better to have fewer, but more powerful tools. In order to be able to identify the most effective training processes, you must also understand how to prioritize. You must learn how to find an application that will enrich your top priority fitness domains and keep others. How do you measure your work capacity? What about your endurance, strength, and power? Where can I start? Let's explore TB's three-pronged strategy. For the first time, we will be doing very little base construction. Fourteen days' aerobic work, endurance, general endurance, or endurance. This could be step 1, or "Block 1" for many trainees, no matter what their ultimate goal. You should also consider your aerobic and strength capabilities, such as the ability to heat water. You create large reservoirs and then dip into them to build subcategories including strength-endurance, anaerobic force, and also the rest. The more you can dig into your well, the more raw material is available to improve your other abilities. To illustrate, training maximal strength at a high level allows you to build a stronger threshold for strength endurance. If you have a high level SE, your SE will push you further than someone with a lower level. One guy may do 100 push ups, while the other man might do 50. If you draw too much water, the well may eventually run dry. You can see this when you begin teaching strength-endurance or high repeat bodyweight. This happens if you do too much long-term work. Your maximum potency levels begin to decrease and you become less effective. As the time passes, strength endurance decreases. You ever wonder why doing a lot more push ups over time doesn't work after a few weeks? Then, your strength-endurance drops. You may need to return to max resistance training temporarily. This reservoir should be topped up. Similar principles apply to anaerobic and aerobic techniques. It is crucial to remember that Block inch should never be overlooked. We will build you a more powerful, larger petrol tank as well as a high-performance engine. Your brain may benefit from a higher threshold. This period will gradually help you get used to working longer hours and can open the door for more intense potential training. Another negative effect that endurance training can have, although it is not often discussed, is the hardening of your mind and raising your tolerance for pain. It can encourage perseverance and help you to keep going. You will find that stage protocol is not too overwhelming once you have gone through overload I. If you skip overload I and just go back to your conditioning program, you might end up hurting more and maybe not growing as much at the end. You can trust the process. We will have some guidelines that we follow throughout the period. These can help increase your motivation to exercise. This cube is slightly more straight-forward and elastic than what your next protocol will be. It was created to help you get the foundations in place for more advanced training. These domain names are foundational to physical fitness. The further you can go, the more time you have. The further you have the further you're able to form additional'secondary' features. After you've completed base construction, choose a continuation template/protocol that suits your needs. It is possible to modify this routine with the various workout sessions available at Working out Vault, Section II, and other publications. You will also learn how to blend your conditioning protocols with your preexisting strength program. The end product will be your strength and conditioning regimen. This course will teach you how to increase your energy levels and market and program several physical fitness domains. Base-building will allow you to see your own conditioning protocol. Measure two could be the exact conditioning protocol.

Why asset training

Common strategy to lose weight is to perform a lot of rowing activities, including distance running, biking, swimming, and cycling. But it is not always an effective strategy. Being a fitness expert, it is obvious that an isolated aerobics training program isn't the best way to shed weight. For the best weight loss results, weight training should be included in your overall weight loss plan. Many people believe that resistance training should be used for muscle building and toning. It is wrong. Even though resistance training doesn't help with weight loss, the profits are under-estimated. Here are reasons weight training should be integrated into your weight loss programs.

Metabolic Rate

Between 24 and 48 hours, weight training was shown to increase metabolic rate after exercise. A high metabolism process allows the body to burn fat more quickly than in rest. Therefore, your body won't just burn fat during exercise; it will also be more efficient at burning fat during rest and sleep.

Encourages Lean Muscle Mass Mass

If you row a lot, it is possible to lose your muscles. You can avoid this by practicing proper training.

Faster Muscle

Training will increase your muscle density, which in turn will lead to a faster metabolic process. This is because muscles are more metabolically intensive than carbs. Simply put, muscle requires more energy to burn than carbs. The result is that more muscle means more calories are burned off.

Reduced training time

In addition to a faster metabolic process induced by resistance training, your system becomes more efficient in burning fat in the rest. This means that you don't have need to focus on burning extra fat by rowing. You can reduce the amount of time you train and see greater weight loss.

Many men and women don't see the value in working out and are worried about what other training options might do to their bodies. Your body will burn fat more quickly if you train it. This will make it less difficult to get on the treadmill, and may also help you to be more active. The ideal resistance training course or supplement program must be set up for the patient to achieve the best results.

It is obvious that exercise has many benefits. These include weight loss, weight maintenance, decreased body fat, improved lungs, heart health, more energy, and reduced chances of developing cardiovascular disease. These benefits are endless. The best thing for many health conditions is exercise.

Because I survived in Columbus Ohio for the past 2-3 years, I now recognize another benefit to standard training and staying well. Los Angeles allows you to become more physically active and motivated for exercise. It will be sunny almost every day of the season, and also the daily temperatures will often reach the 70's or 80's. This afternoon, the most important weather decision you need to make is whether or not you will be wearing the brownish and gloomy pants. Everyone is back in LA running, biking, walking and playing golf. Hollywood All Things Considered.

This is Columbus, my home. While you may have your ardent physical fitness enthusiasts (me included-you could take the girl in LA but you cannot manhunter this girl), there are many others who venture out, regardless of the weather. They are often found outside on the roads, running, walking or cross-country skiin the playground (yes I did see a girl achieve this the other day), and walking their dogs in snow, ice, or winter. Others are content to stay at home and not have the energy to go to the gym, elliptical or exercise bike.

Most people find it difficult to get moving or have the energy to do any exercise. It is possible that you are not aware of how energy works. The longer you work, the more energy your body may have. The reason is that exercise increases blood circulation, oxygen, and energy. This gives you a great feeling of high and natural happiness. What could possibly be better?

I can agree that these few months of winter can be exhausting emotionally. Being able to survive the summer in the Midwest is no easy feat. It is even more challenging to be healthy and fit. To wash your car and not let it freeze, shovel snow when it's too cold, and then walk into the snow and ice to look at the vehicle. It takes much more to get yourself packed up and ready to go. There are so many people who fall and slip and injure themselves and they fear going out. This is why routine exercise and resistance training are important.

Strength-training creates a MindBody link, so you can be in tune to your own body. While you should be paying attention to the muscles you are exercising, you must also pay attention to how your body feels. Strength training encourages you to "tune into your own body", since it focuses on endurance, stamina, and endurance. There's no doubt that weight training is something everyone should do at least two to three days each week. It is never too late to get started. There are numerous studies that show it to be the best method to lose weight. You'll feel better.

Strengthening the muscles of the joints is a great way to prevent the damage that ordinary people, athletes, and sport fans often suffer from those same muscles repeatedly. Also, you can improve your balance while strength training. This will allow you to navigate around the everyday, including in the arctic, snowy parking lots, and roads.

It is obvious that exercise has many benefits. These include weight loss and maintenance, decreased body fat, improved lungs, heart health, more energy, lessening your chances of developing cardiovascular disease, and making it easier to feel great on your own. These benefits are endless. The best thing for many health conditions is exercise.

Because I survived in Columbus Ohio for the past 2-3 years, I now recognize another benefit to standard training and staying well. Los Angeles allows you to become more physically active and motivated for exercise. It will be sunny almost every day of the season and the daily temperatures are usually in the 70s or 80s. This afternoon, the most important weather decision you need to make is whether or not to wear the dark brown shorts and the grey shorts. Everyone else is busy in LA running, biking, walking and golfing. Hollywood All Things Considered.

This is Columbus, my home. While you may have your ardent physical fitness enthusiasts (me included, you can simply take the girl in LA but you cannot manhunter this girl), there are many others who brave the elements no matter what the weather. They can be seen running, walking, skiing cross country in the playground (yes that was a girl who achieved this feat), and walking their dogs, as they navigate through the snow, ice or winter. Other people are content to stay at home and not have the energy to go to the gym, elliptical or exercise bike.

However, many people find it extremely difficult to get moving or have the energy to do any kind of exercise. It is possible that you are not aware that energy. The longer you do something the more energy may be available to you. It is because when you work out and exercise, you can not only boost blood circulation and oxygen in the human brain and muscles but you also release endorphins that provide an all natural high. This gives you a wonderful sensation. What could possibly be better?

I can agree that these few months of winter can be exhausting emotionally. Being able to survive the summer in the Midwest is no easy feat. It is also more challenging than ever to be healthy and fit. It will require energy, strength, balance and strength to wash the car and shovel snow. It takes much more to get yourself packed up and ready to go. There are so many people who fall and slip, and then injure themselves, that they fear going out. This is why regular exercise and resistance training are essential.

Strength training can help you feel more connected to your body. While doing exercises, you should be thinking about the muscles you may be working out. Strengthtraining encourages you to "listen" to your body while you focus on improving your stamina as well as endurance. Resistance training is something that everyone should do at least two to three times each week. It is not too late to start. Studies show it is the most effective way to shed excess weight. You'll look and feel better.

Strengthening your joints would be the perfect way to avoid the many harms that athletes, fans and everyone else who uses these muscles often face. Also, you can improve your balance while strength training. This will aid you in your everyday tasks such as driving on snowy roads and parking lots.

Every girl will at one point in her lives look to reduce her weight. Men are also affected by the same issues, although at a less severe level. No matter what sexual activity you engage in, weight loss is possible if you stop eating ordinary food. The other side of this coin is that it is vital to keep an eye on how many calories you are consuming. Also, it is crucial to have the right mix and combination of exercises that will aid your weight loss efforts as well as tone your muscles.

It is easy to overlook the importance of building muscles when we start a fat-loss program. It is possible to combine all your efforts towards losing weight with exercises that will build muscle, which can make you feel better. Studies have shown that more muscles equals more calories burned per day. You can achieve this beautiful toned body by doing resistance training.

My experience has shown that many girls do not incorporate resistance training exercises into their fitness programs. You could have looked at pictures of body builders, and seen the slender and rippling muscles they had achieved by lifting weights. You won't be able to conquer Ms. Olympia if you don't lose some pounds. You may not achieve the body of a female Olympic athlete if your hormones aren't in place. This means you will have to spend hours strength training male coworkers at the office. It's not necessary to incorporate weights into your intensity training exercises. You will not only lose the weight but your body will be toned and envy-worthy. You might find it not too bad, I'm sure.

You are looking for resistance training exercises to help you reach your goals. Going to the gym at your community could be a great place to begin. It's possible to talk to a variety of physical fitness professionals about the best ways to slim down, gain muscle, and tone your body. Many fitness professionals will be delighted to help you with your workouts and diet plans. It is as simple as running with a 100ml jar. This will help build muscles. Your arms will look amazing after you do your cardio vascular exercises. You might also be able to lift 2Lb dumbbells. It's possible to have fun with your workouts. You may also be able to build muscle mass by using chunks. There is no need to be a slave to your body in pursuit of building it. It is actually much simpler than you may think.

Another fantastic place to find strength training activities is online. You must ensure that your surroundings are free of clutter and prone to any items that could lead to injury or death for you or others. Do not lift any weights that are causing strain to your muscles. Negligence of your surroundings and following the body's reaction when you lift weights can lead to serious injury to the body. It is easy to see the appeal of weight training. If you do it for a few minutes each week, you might notice impressive results that will attract envious glances from both friends and foes.

I will let you know a little bit about a key. To get the best shape possible, you need to mix strength-training and running. Many people ignore strength training because of ignorance, or because they see it as a means to gain muscle and not to lose body weight. In this article I will show you the benefits of weight training.

The American College of Sports Medicine suggests that adults do a few strength exercises each week. You will be a far more efficient jogger if you have stronger muscles. Running is much easier when your whole body is strong. You can run faster if your torso is strong.

Studies have shown that a strong heart (stomach/back) can help absorb shock from running. Running is all about your thighs. It is possible to decrease the amount of jolt they use, which will increase their efficiency over the long-term.

This is not a discussion about major strength training. It's not my goal to make you look like a professional body builder. It is not the goal to tone or firm your body. I highly recommend that weight training be added to your running schedule in the coming weeks. I believe you will enjoy the way this system feels and looks.

We will be discussing the reasons resistance training is more effective than aerobic fat burning in this Guide. A majority of people are mistakenly under the impression that cardio is the easiest and most effective way to lose weight and gain muscle. This was shown to be wrong. Resistance training strengthens muscles and increases metabolism, which helps to burn off fat. The more muscles you have the easier it is to lose fat. Any weight loss program must include some form of weight training. It is not necessary to have a gym membership. Many workouts are possible without the use of weights or any other equipment.

Cardio-exercises work well for warming your body and getting blood flowing. However if your goal is to burn fat, resistance training should be part of your fitness plan. Weight loss requires some form of intensity training. Because weight loss lifting increases muscle tissue, which in turn increases metabolism and burns fat. Some very basic exercises to reduce your body weight, like pushups and squats for the human body, are possible. These are only two types of weight training that can be used to reduce weight. They target your torso and legs as well as your gluts. Larger muscles also burn more calories than those with smaller muscle groups.

You should take only ten minutes each morning to do push-ups and weight squats. There is no need for weights. It is important to perform weight training exercises slowly, so you do not get fatigued. As an example, once you've completed a pushup and are at the floor, slow down and count to 10. Then, move slowly upwards into the number 10. Continue this process until you're unable to do more pushups. For human body weight squats, use the same technique. You can start with 10 reps. Pause at the base to perform another rep. Then, gradually increase your speed to reach the count of 10. Continue this process until you are exhausted. This technique can improve endurance and increase fat burning capacity. It also reduces the risks of injury from quick jerking motions.

A weight training program is essential for fat reduction. This is not something you can achieve with just cardio. Resistance training can be great for the heart. It requires your own heart pump to work harder. You can strengthen your heart by training it harder.

Why is Bar Bell so special?

Guilt is something that people can feel a lot of at one time or another, especially in the context of exercise. Being able to hold a barbell and using it often will help you overcome the guilt that growing waistlines and weight could lead to.

A workout routine at home can be a good way to get rid of obesity. In fact, you can use it as part of your exercise program. Everyone can get fitter by avoiding some of the conditions that being overweight may lead to. All you need is some time and energy. One step towards the ideal goal is to purchase one of those many Olympic barbell collection.

You should consider a number of things when choosing to exercise at your home. Safety is of paramount importance. A barbell can be set up to provide safety for those who train in your home. It is important to consider the location of your basement or garage. Concrete floors are the best option for these areas. Barbell places, which can be kept in the basement or garage and take up little space when not in use, can be kept easily.

There is always going to be disagreement. You can train at your home, or you can join a gym in your neighborhood. Due to rising health costs and the need to coach multiple people at once, a one hour workout may quickly turn into two hours at your gym. There's privacy and relaxation in the home. You don't have to wait for anyone to finish before you can shoot your turn. A cap barbell, Olympic or Olympic weight barbell can help you exercise at a much more enjoyable place whenever you have enough free time. The benefits of exercising at home have been proven to be helpful in fat loss.

Olympic barbell collections can help a person be confident they are using the correct equipment. The best training is based on the information. A Cap or Olympic rib will give you a better workout than any other exercise center.

It's a smart idea to have multiple tees or barbell bars for most instruction programs. This makes it much easier to do a workout. It reduces the need to shift the weights onto the bar and eliminates interruptions that can affect endurance.

Anyone who powertrains can reap the benefits from picking up a barbell sooner or later.

Barbells make it easier to perform rotational motions such squats, deadlifts or squats. Lauren Pak (a NASM-certified trainer and cofounder Attain Fitness Boston) tells SELF. Barbells can be manipulated with ease by its weight plates. Barbells could be the best way to grow and maintain your weight.

It is important to know that you need to grab a barbell. However, upcoming a single exercise with Optimism and knowing that you need to grab a barbell are two different things. Chase Karnes (C.S.C.S.S.S.) is a Kentucky-based strength & conditioning pro. "Whenever I look at a lifter who's new to barbell, then they seem somewhat shy, cloudy and overwhelmed," he says. "It is perfectly normal and part to getting out of your routine."

Chapter 2: How To Know If You Should Prepare For Barbells

To You can begin using barbells. There's no time limit on how much you should train. Rather the only thing that is 100 percent mandatory is excellent kind, Anna Swisher Ph.D.C.S.S., USA Weightlifting's trainer education director and sport science chief, tells SELF. It is essential to be able do basic movements with your own leg and kettlebells.

Pak asserts that you should feel comfortable with the softball pressing, pressing and hinging functions of the deadlift, bench, squat and deadlift from the moment your reach a barbell.

These are some samples of progressions you could use to get to barbells. Once you're able to perform each one with great form, you can incorporate Bar Bell variations of this movement into your daily routine.

Progressions: single-arm overhead barbell press, Double-arm overhead barbell press (displayed here), single-arm over-head kettle bell media, double-arm over-head kettle bell media

If you're working with barbells to get to grips, it is also important to think about how free your joints are when doing any given exercise. Pak states that Barbells restrict movement. He suggests that you adjust to the Bar Bell.

To take an example, in order to place your back into a good back-squat, you will need your shoulder and back free to receive your hands behind your mind, without straining your spine. Pak states that deadlifts must be done in a way that hinges your buttocks, while maintaining a neutral spine as you lower to ground. If you are forced to bend your spine to get to the pub, then you should work on trendy mobility before you attempt barbell deadlifts. You might do better pulling or pushing if your shoulders are hurting. Your muscles don't necessarily have the same symmetry, so it is possible that they are ordered in a way which allows them to follow a similar movement trail.

Swisher also says, "If you recognize that you have a complex injury history or suffer pain with specific movements, you will absolutely want to help a trainer to start."

The different types of barbells

When you are deciding to begin using barbells, it is important to assess your strength. You will find a variety of barbells, so it is possible to find one that works best for you.

The Olympic Rib, the most popular barbell in fitness centres, is a barbell that you will find in most electricity racks. It weighs about 4-5 pounds (20 kg). Swisher stated that this barbell can be used to do exercises such squats, presses, and other similar movements. She also suggested that weight plates could be added to each side to aid in fat loss. "If the one you have is too thick then check to see if there is a smaller one."

There are lighter options, such as a women's Olympic Pub that weighs 35 pounds (1-5 Kilogram). It is smaller than other Olympic pubs and has a larger diameter. This makes them easier for you to grasp once you have the hands on. You may find fixed or preloaded barbells convenient (such as that one). They are smaller and easier for you to reach, and some weigh only 3-5 lbs.

Pre-loaded barbells work well for exercises such as overhead Presses and shoulder curls. However they don't always perform well for principal powerlifts such squats, bench presses, and deadlifts," Pak states. He thinks they are too short to be able to compete with safety-bar-clad powerstands. Pre-loaded barbells make dead-lifting difficult. The plates are usually smaller so you need to drop far enough to select the bar. This could lead to form problems. It is important to use rubberized bumper plate on one side when dead-lifting. These plates are the exact same height as the barbell, so no matter what your weight, you won't ever have to go insanely low to reach it.

The last, many health clubs offer snare bars. These bars are also called hex pubs. You will need to use one and stand at the center of it. These pubs have a weight plate on each side and change in fat. This is because the pub's weight is distributed around the front, so many individuals can lift more weight with a snare than they could with an Olympic pub. Although they appear complicated, they are completely beginner-friendly.

How to use barbell racks

Pak stated that "one the most difficult things from the Start" is "putting the Racks in place." This is because each fitness center has slightly different options, making it difficult to give clear instructions on how to do it properly.

The most commonly used contraptions when holding barbells include submersible racks as well as electricity Stands. In the above photo, the squatrack is at the rear while the energy rack is to the top. They'll have weight hooks that can be placed on the pub to rest when not being used, along with safety bars and hooks that can be grabbed if you shed the pub charge. These pub hooks are usually flexible and fit in the holes on the rack framework. Ask a trainer, personal trainer, or a fitness professional if you need help with your problem. Karnes says that even veterans sometimes have difficulty with power or squat racks. Therefore, you shouldn't feel ashamed.

Your ranges of motion should be considered when setting up the elevation at which the barbell and security pubs can be placed.

Swisher points out that if you're squatting you need to do it within the ability shelf with all the pubs just below your bottom. "This will enable you to lower the pub below the basic safety bar and then you can continue the reps.

Another important security trick is to keep your weight under control. The pub has weight clips that can be attached immediately. They come in many forms like metal bands or plastic collars. Therefore, Pak advises that if you have difficulty with them, it's not a shame to ask for help. The clips can be found inside the weight racks and in a bin close to the barbells.

Some health clubs may also have electricity and jet racks. It is usually easy to use this barbell, but it can be difficult to move in an unnatural or also dangerous manner due to the predetermined course. If you are looking for a completely free way to lose fat, this is the place to go. You can use this in cases where a physical therapist or personal trainer tells you to exercise in a safe environment. Or if you're unable to make a barbell work for you. Cool thrusts are one example.

Remember, Smith machines usually weigh significantly less than bars (usually 1520 lbs), and your system doesn't have to work as hard to stabilize the pub while you exercise. This means that you may lift more weight on a Smith machine then you would with a barbell.

There are many methods to maintain a barbell.

There are many different ways to hold a Barbell. It all depends on the purpose of your practice and the type and brand of Bar Bell you are using.

Pronated. This grip is the most frequent way to raise a barbell. This grip isn't the strongest and can limit how much weight you can carry during exercises like deadlifts.

Supinated. This clasp is a place where your palms are up. It's also great for curls and row variants, in which you want to target the biceps. It will not perform well with additional barbell exercises.

Alternated: This involves holding the Bar Bell with one hand at a pronated and one at a sucpinated grip. This allows you more weight than is possible with a double hand grip. This may increase the risk of hammering your biceps knees or knees. It is best to alternate the way you place each hand for each pair. This will ensure equal work for both arms.

Twist: This involves grasping the bar with pronated hands. But, together with the palms curving across the hands and a pronated grip. The clasp is capable of assisting you to lift heavier loads at deadlifts. It is most commonly used in Pilates contests. You should only use it when necessary.

Neutral: Holding the barbells in a neutral position with your hands on is not possible. It can be used, but only when using trap/hex pubs. This is an ideal position to use for people with stiff shoulders.

Accessory such as lifting and straps

Take a look at your Gym Goers who are using barbells. They will likely have a lot of paraphernalia like gloves and straps.

Karnes states, "Gifts can be a fantastic option if your palms are very dry." However, in order to prevent calluses, it is best to use straps or to lift au naturel.

He clarified that straps typically function to Help You hold bars that are greater than your hands can support. The lifting straps will help you lift more weight and not place as much strain on your chest.

Pak does NOT recommend straps that are too heavy or for beginners. They are "just Going to be More Useful in the Event that You are Already Very Mesmerized by the Practice and You Are Just Using Them For This Last Little Advantage," she says.

Like all strength coaching, it involves controlling the Bar Bell Staples. It may take just one of the furthest steps, with no additional bells and whistles.

Why Barbells Are Far Better Than Machines

The first thing a person does when they walk into a fitness facility is to be confused about where to invest their Timing.

Let's clarify it: Bar Bell coaching will teach you how to Teach For Your Advantage. No other. Bar Bell Exercises, presses or dead-lifts are unrivaled in their power and ability to increase strength, muscle size, power, and power. The rationale barbells are therefore very valuable is they are definitely the most ergonomically-friendly load-handling tool in life -- they also allow very heavyweights to become gripped from the hands and proceeded directly across the middle of their foot. Barbells' flexibility allows for small stresses to be placed on the entire human body by using the entire range of flexibility available to your main grip systems. These small increases can add up to astonishing increases in size, strength, and endurance that can last many years.

For a long time, fitness centers were built with barbells. It was pretty much what you brought to a fitness centre to use -- a metal pub and iron plates that were inserted to help with weight loss. You can perform a limited number of exercises if you use them while standing with one foot on the soil. To do this, you might place the pub on your stomach or back, then squat and stand straight up. It could be placed in your hands, and you can push it up. You can also set it in your hands, push it up and then pick it up. These basic approaches worked well because they combined the average actions from all your muscles, joints, and bones.

Bar-Bell Training Works - Fighting Gravity

A good way to describe reputation barbell training is to: follow your Body mass as well as a weighted blbell at a vertical position along your centre. The midst of your foot. Gravity plays a major role in the movement's power. Amazingly, gravity operates in one direction: right down. In other words, the way that you constantly work against gravity cannot be any other than right up. Your body will naturally balance in the middle of your feet if you adopt a straight position, similar to when lifting heavy loads. It is usually true that the best way to lift lots of weight is very close to the body. This would mean you should be able to lift the maximum amount of weight in the vertical direction upwards. This is easier than with oddly-shaped equipment like lawnmowers.

Your normal way to manage any loading would be to keep the pounds near your entire body. This is how you do it without thinking about it. Think about the next time you pick up something heavy from the floor. You will burst as close as you can to it. Your experience has shown that the lighter the load is, the easier it would be for you to lift. Chances are, that if you get hurt while trying to handle your lawnmower, it was because the load wasn't balanced enough.

Barbell coaching changed dramatically with the increased usage of different kinds and types of chairs. The seat press was able to displace the standard press, while the UpperBody exercise in the gymnasium was kept simple. Benches allow the guts and balance to be transferred onto your back or buttocks. That is how the seat presses or other seated Squat exercises function. Bar-Bell training calls for a default posture, which is a position that places all the strain on the feet and distributes the weight equally under the body.

The Bar-Bell offers a way to add weight to your body's daily movements. It is a course that essentially makes your system stronger, whether it wishes to or not. It is possible to lift 175lbs if you start with a 45-pound Bar Bell. You are as high as 305 in a calendar year. Even though you start with just 4-5 lbs, almost no body is as strong as that of your mom. She may have even had to take your grumbling feet off the ground for all those years.

Barbell coaching has many advantages: it is straightforward, logical, efficient, cost-effective, and, most importantly, reliable. It has been used in its original form for many decades by a large number of people. Additionally, it has served as the strength-training platform for athletes since the beginning of 20th century. It is not surprising that modern fitness centers contain machines, rather than just weights and dumbbells.

You Create a Fresh Business

Alternative methods to becoming stronger include making use of a collection of odds and ends, which were found in gyms owned or managed by men who may weld. These machines could function with several muscles simultaneously. Some of the older photographs of leg extension and leg curling machines can be seen in magazines that date back to the 50s and 60s.

Arthur Jones started marketing his Nautilus Line to all levels of the fitness industry, including high schools, universities, colleges and high schools. Their beautifully designed, elegantly constructed electric blue machines were sold in just two years. Nautilus revolutionized gym business by creating the concept for the modern gymnasium. This is the same one that you are likely to be part of, with sales offices at the front, large rooms full of glowing machines, and many employees floating the ground.

The articular Circuit consists of 12 exercises. Each exercise is performed in its own sequence. You have destroyed it. You will be raped. Fried/barbequed/blasted/obliterated/murdere d you. The articular circuit humbled the once-haughty high school athlete. It did not make anyone stronger than any other thing, aside from Nautilus machine, which worked for approximately 6 weeks. A person who has been trained will find that any such thing works for approximately 6 weeks. However, if you are a newbie to a physical job, it will cause adaptation which will make you stronger. For Around 6 months.

Nautilus was simple to operate, manage and train, both from a company standpoint. This is exactly why the Nautilus Club version was so popular: the company had not invested in training or exercise, but on the earnings. An employer may hire anyone who wants to be a "trainer" at a machine-based gym. This took approximately 3-5 mins. Because there aren't any variations, it is not necessary to know how adjust the chair height. You might then spend your money on earnings staff training. This makes sense from an control perspective.

Additionally, the machine-based clubs version gave rise to a new strategy in the rapidly expanding market for university degrees in physical education. As PE scholars were working and health clubs were forming, the machine-based practice model was slowly adopted by the academic community. It was the use of exercise machines that allowed us to study the individual body's response and reaction to stress, which contributed greatly to the creation of a peer-reviewed human body of literature.

The past few decades have witnessed a fascinating position, even though more people than ever in history are diligently exercising. However, most do this poorly. Machine-based exercise does not work well, and it is crucial that you understand the reasons.

Why Machines don't Work

It may appear that you are not physically capable of making yourself stronger by doing something challenging. Strength is the most popular physiological adaptation because it has a positive effect on all the other bodily features. Strong people are more than just their quadriceps, biceps and waist.

Since machines don't have the ability to support this aggressive strength-athlete's Program, they aren't able to. They operate like motors, operating the levers throughout the entire skeleton. That's how we all strike the heaps every day if we use our own bodies. While machines use only a few levers at once, the deadlift employs many. These may all work together and might help to move more weight than two of them.

Barbells can be used to put more strain on your body than one vertical muscle. While the ability to cause physical discomfort if a muscle group is isolated is possible, the muscle's capacity to produce force is limited by its bulk. This limits its ability to increase stamina. Dead lifts and exercises like presses are able to produce more potency adaptation and worry about muscle density than is the case with isolation exercises.

Many machines, as we have already mentioned, can choose to operate a couple muscles at a given time and only one or two joints. It's easy to spot the problem with them: they don't work enough to build enough muscle tissue to generate enough general stress to make such a change. They can be worked hard enough to make you feel as bad as they are, but they won't make your life easier or more productive. Use strength is more important than movement around an individual congregated. Crunches can make you strong, while leg extensions won't.

All Fall-down

Some machines require more muscle and joints, like Hammer Strength Football Market apparatus. A few machines, including the Smith Machine in the majority of modern nightclubs may even look like barbells. One common characteristic of all exercise machines will not allow them to collapse as you use them.

This seemingly insignificant detail is important. Normal individual motion -- the condition under which our bodies are used to interact with our environment every day -- can be very complex. It's the result of the collective efforts of thousands of muscles moving many visceral components, all under the supervision of 1000s and more nerves. You can't just balance your weight across your feet daily, which is an ever-more difficult job for the older and frailer population. But every thing you do requires the coordinated interplay between one's stamina along with its mass.

It is important to learn how to manipulate the barbell within your body's normal movement range. Employing one's knees (or hips), back, wrists (or elbows), wrists (or wrists), and all the muscles that move them together under extremely heavy loads -- keeping vertical ensures that your joints as well your muscles work just like they were designed to: increasing strength while maintaining balance.

In addition, the ability to use power in place of imbalance is a key part of daily life and sports. Field strength is the ability to exert tremendous force even when your body has lost its balance. This is why it was called "field strength". The best way to increase strength is by working equally at two feet. This is because that's where the weight might be increased. It is important to have the ability to perform in low-than-optimal positions for field sports as well as life. The ability to accomplish tasks without being balanced can be increased by increasing your strength.

The System Should Move in the Right Way

For server exercisers, it is even more important to consider the constrained, artificial movement patterns that are imposed upon them by this gadget. A standard way for legs to function would be for knees to extend and bend in a coordinated manner. Agonists as well as antagonists work simultaneously. Hamstrings have quads, quads, calves and other fashionable muscles all work together. This includes squats and deadlifts, walking, running and even running. It is not smart to sit on a system while your buttocks are pulled down at the chair with both your hands joined, or bend your elbows as your upper arms and shoulders remain motionless. It is a recipe for overuse injuries. Since one joint presses against another, causing ligaments and other tendons to perform tasks they were not designed for, it is really a dumb way to sit. Arthur Jones's Nautilus System through Arthur's Idea of the Ideal Movement to Get an Isolated Muscle Band falls woefully short of decent physical preparation, for both sports and life.

The ability to produce force against an immune system outside of your body may be what gives power its name. There's only one kind of strength. It is the strength that your muscles produce from the components of the skeletal system. These connect to the floor using items that you hold with your hands. Building strength will ensure that you have increased your skill to create force. This means that you must use heavier weights. The use of machines to accomplish this is not only inefficient, but also because of the inherent nature of isolation exercise.

Chapter 3: Key To Success

To understand success, it is important to know what it means. This is the first step towards success. The best definition that I have come across is: "Success means you complete what you set out to do." To put it another way, success means completing the task you set out.

Even approving a Bank is a Sort Of Success if that was all you had. But you probably didn't want to end up in prison.

The above definition of Achievements shines a spotlight on both success and failure. Follow the steps and you will be successful. Don't try to follow along with others if you don't have an idea.

This provides a yardstick to help people estimate the daily events in their lives. At the end, we can declare that "I have neglected" or "I have won"

This may sound obvious, but it is quite amazing that only 85 percent end up doing exactly what they intended.

I asked many people what success looked like. One man said "Success involves making lots of money." Another person stated that success is about "achieving your goals." Someone else suggested that victory was about "strengthening you potential". Another interesting answer was that winning is "Earning what others want".

Brian Tracy Will Seek All the Connections between Goals and Success He stated that success will be achieved by setting goals and commenting on them. Tracy believes that those who set clear goals are more likely to achieve their goals in a shorter period of time than people who do not.

Stuart Goldsmith from "The Midas Method" has an important section on the best way to create goals, so they can be achieved by using the entire power of their sub conscious minds.

Maria Nemeth is a great example of the respect of achievement. "Doing what you say you will do, with ease."

Nearly every race, except politicians, is unable to do what they said they would. To do it effortlessly, you need to be able to use the sub conscious mind.

Jim Rohn says that there are only a couple of straightforward disciplines you can practice every day to achieve success.

The Ability of Everyday area has huge potential. Each day, the results are cumulative. This incredible practice is performed 365 days per year with perhaps a few lapses.

It is not difficult to have enormous influence. When the subject becomes an everyday routine, it can be easily forgotten about and lost.

A writer who writes daily has written at least 300 pages by season's end. If they stop writing, they lose their motivation and momentum. Writing should be done daily, but only a few lines per day. This will help you attract the right thoughts.

One of the American press students from Liverpool was recently employed in 600 occupations. He received only 1 interview. He decided to make a book. He performed ten pages each morning. He performed at night in a desperate attempt to raise money. After that, he composed until the early hours of the morning in the famous publication. It also reminds you of learning to star in a Hollywood blockbuster.

He mentions that the Event That You Write 1 Page per Day for 100 Days is enough to create a screenplay. He began by studying the structure of 2 other books. He discovered the order in which they were placed. Then he wrote his screenplay after analyzing film footage and finding out how long each scene lasted.

I do not remember his title or Name of the publication, as I only knew a part of it on TV.

One can completely change their lives by establishing a custom of daily areas. The best thing about daily areas is their ability to create customs. Customs can also create personality.

Jim Ryun, American Athlete is great at the following:

"Motivation gives you the drive to keep going.

Habit is what keeps us moving.

Another incredible quote would be:

"Do not try to become a successful person; instead, strive to be an individual of value."

Albert Einstein

The following quote says it all:

Henry David Thoreau

Many will claim that achievement doesn't mean making money. It is about being a valuable person.

But, this can lead to making money. People are able to cover important. If a person is skilled at their profession, they can often choose what type of coverage they would like.

Adam Hollioake is a successful British county cricket captain. After Ben, his younger brother was killed in an automobile accident in Perth Australia, he realized just what is important in life. Adam learned that it was important to be kind and generous to those who enjoy life.

His vision of cricket success would be not always winning. He doesn't mind dropping a game of cricket. He doesn't mind if his team does not put in 100% effort. He comments:

"When you set that goal, you Usually win anyway."

You must put in 100 percent effort for all outcomes to achieve success. It is more common than not that the result will be exceptional.

Michael Angier provides a brilliant definition of succeeding.

Gradually working towards our important objectives is the key to success. When we put all our energy and efforts on the things that matter, we cannot help but succeed.

Angier also admires Ralph Waldo Emerson's remarks about achievement.

To have fun often and often; gain the respect of intelligent individuals and the affection of kids;

and yet, make the appreciation for honest critics and suffer the betrayal from false friends; to love beauty and discover the best; yet, make the world a bit better, no matter how healthy a child is or what social situation they are in; to realize that every life you have lived has been easier because of your experiences; this truly is to have succeeded.

What causes success and what causes collapse?

William James, the Fantastic American Psychologist, says failure is caused by insufficient faith at 1 self

"Human collapsing is only possible if there's one cause." It's the lack of faith in one's true self.

Faith in your own ability to succeed is a huge part of success. Stuart Goldsmith talks about two types or beliefs that can help you achieve success. You need to believe in yourself and be able to do so.

Substance is yet another source of great success.

Brian Tracy says that the key to success is "the ability to delay gratification in short term in order to receive greater rewards over time"

Another reason is your openness to win if success seems distant.

"Far away, in the sunlight are My greatest ambitions. While I may not reach them, I will see beauty, believe in it and try to follow them wherever they lead.

Louisa May Alcott (1832-1888) American Author

Danny, my personal computer expert, thinks that you should keep a fantasy going in all situations and not move forward. If you feel like giving up, use an ironfist to capture your vision.

Danny has had a dream for over 22 decades. His fantasy is for the world to have the best languages translator.

No matter your age, you can still live the dream. You can really imagine yourself achieving this dream. Too many women and men are tired of their lives and give up on their dreams.

Each fantasy is personal, but the Principle is exactly the same. You are an idiot if your release. You have to be committed to a cause. Do not release until you die. Instead, set yourself a goal.

There's nothing you can't do. If you cannot swim 10 feet without stopping, train for at least a month and you will soon be able swim 50 feet.

Danny's comments regarding swimming made me realize how little I was taught about the benefits of training.

The annual half mile swim from the ocean was part of my college experience on the Isle of Man. I knew I would drown when I tried that but no one ever suggested I begin exercising to make it possible.

I was classified as someone who could not perform the swim. It never occurred to me that after ascertained training, I would be able complete exactly what was impossible for me previously.

Danny was a small, weakling child when he grew up. One afternoon, he realized this wasn't a good thing. He completed and did a bit of weight training, and set his own fitness, flexibility and power goals.

This is what he does every single day. This prevents him from becoming bored with his everyday routine. He can do 200 situps. 30-50 leg increases. Four or three collections are available of 20-30 seat press.

He performs 20- or 30-minute sets of dumbell exercises to increase his leg strength. You won't be able to balance with dumb-bells. There are also very few chances that you'll lose weight with your kids or loved ones. Dumbells are more controllable than barbells.

Danny would advise you to always perform Something. Study a publication if you're not sure. The best thing you can do is to lay down and watch TV. You can choose to do this, and nothing will happen. He also mentions the hypnotic influence television has on audiences. Danny barely watches television.

Danny is also amazed that Arnold Schwarzenegger has been elected Governor in California. Arnold is a person who will only do what is necessary to obtain something. He would eat 50 mars pubs every time he was required to. He was able to bear being naked for half an hour in a field.

This is a great example. To send your email sales letter, you don't have to put stamps on tens or thousands of envelopes.

The principle of the universe is that you must do what is necessary. Some issues require specific activities to reach them, and you must do them regardless of whether or not you are enjoying them.

Although I may say that I Need Army of California, I do not want to go on public speaking tours or travel about campaign trails or be more friendly to tens of millions of people you don't like. It is necessary to grab babies and smile at people who are not like you.

These ideas will make you wealthy if you wish to be rich. It doesn't make any sense to say "I don't really want to do it" Danny gives himself an electronic smack when he's tempted to give up his endeavours.

Many people think that they can make a lot of money by simply suing people or fraud. The world would be a much better place if people did exactly what they were supposed to do.

Many successful women and men worry about the importance of being active in order to be successful.

Michael Masterson writes in this E Zine entitled "Early to Rise". He says that action is key to success and failure to act is why many people will never achieve the kind of success they wish for.

One way to achieve Success is to always remain cool. You can only do the important things and those you enjoy doing.

Sir David Frost: "Do not strive for success if that is what you Desire"

Donna Presley was given information by Elvis Presley to assist her in achieving her dreams for the future. It seemed to me that it was good guidance.

Donna's favorite memory of Elvis is When she was 18, she spoke to him on one. He asked her about her plans in the long term and said that she could do anything.

Elvis had his own Discouragement which he didn't notice. Next was the second part of the life. While not overly impressive, Donna suggested that we should all focus on the amazing things he did.

Peter Vidmar explains his success in the Olympic Games.

"There are just two things I'd like to try and win Olympic silverTrain once, if I had the chance"

This is my favourite quote. It sums up the key to success and the perseverance and discipline required to achieve it. Training may be simple at times but not easy at all the rest of the time. It's very simple and straightforward.

Another one I love is worrying about the type success that is dependent on people liking work or products. It doesn't matter if they want to work. You can do your best to please them or just straighten them up.

"Success can be described as a simple formula: "Do your absolute best so that people can enjoy what you do."

Sam Ewing

Any achievement is not without cost. The next quote usually refers to a boring job. This kind of work is described by the phrase "drudgery". Promotion is an essential part of almost any type business. Most businessmen dislike it.

Drudgery is the key to success. It doesn't come with coercion or bribery. Just pay the purchase amount and it's yours.

Orison Swett Marden, 1850-1924.

Mike Litman frequently includes gold Statements. This is Only One of These:

"The greatest success secret in life is not that you have to be able to do it. All you need is to get it moving. It is possible to lose everything if you are too perfect. We move because we want everything to be perfect. Let us instead, start.

One success breeds another. Bobby Robson, now 70, is not only one of Britain's most successful managers. He must be able to see what is necessary for success. He made the following comment about the performances of his group:

"Success breeds more success"

This is very logical. One publication will make you confident to write another. A novel was written about the suffering of gout by a female aged 70+. It was a huge victory that she was overwhelmed by and earned her thousands and even thousands of dollars. Two books were written about her.

It is an integral goal for many people. But, it will help to clarify what success really means for you. I hope this guide has shed some light on possible definitions and offered ideas on how to achieve your success.

They are considered the benchmark of a healthy and fit individual. It is why their workouts are so envied and desired by non-athletes. It's their disciplined daily routine that makes them stand out from others. Athletes get up in the morning to go to sleep at night. And they leave the comfort of their beds every morning. Maintaining a routine isn't for everyone. You need to be committed and have the drive to reach your highest levels of physical fitness through daily training. This drives athletes to work hard and achieve their goals. What is the most prized and honored goal for these athletes, exactly? They are determined to win the most glory at the Olympic Games, and other world championships regardless of where they come from. The funniest fans of a hard-core work out regimen are the greatest achievers of times. Mark Spitz, Usain bolt, Nadia Comaneci and Mohammad Ali are all examples of the well-organized routines that you have. From following the advice of famous athletes to their daily routine, this report can help you make the transition to wellness and health.

What could be the ideal daily schedule for these athletes? To find the answer to the question, we need to look deeper into the topic. You can still make broad generalizations when you are trying to find the answer. It is because inquirers make the mistake of not identifying other athletic goals. Also, they often link the success, most importantly, to this level fitness degree. While they might have been able to compete at certain sports to an extent, they often fail to recognize that it takes a lot of technical training to attain the desired abilities and strength. Natalie Rizzo, a site writer on nutricisedr.com discussing health, nutrition, and physical fitness, writes in a January blog post about the 2014 Sochi Winter Olympics. We don't always realize that athletes competing in different sports at this Olympics have different goals, which means they need to follow different training and eating regimens. She added, "Some athletes telephone for speed, while other sports focus on power & space." Some athletes get more power from being lean. Others find it helpful to bulk up and improve their power.

Rizzo's study shows there isn't one universal program that works for all athletes. The national and international goals of the athletes determine the disposition of fitness plans. Usain bolt, a sprinter and a shooter-set athlete like Ulf Timmerman or David Storl would follow a completely different daily schedule. It is the players' abilities that determine their practice routine. Usain Blyton, the fastest sprinter on the planet, could be focused on developing training programs that will increase endurance, muscle strength, control breathing, and jumps. Shot Set players will, on the flip, work hard to increase their knee strength, momentum and balance, as well as their ability to throw in a throw ring.

Daily Exercises, Workouts

The technical training for different sports may not be the same, but an individual will learn commonalities from the everyday routine of athletes in all types of sports. The following are some general exercises and workouts athletes might follow closely:

* The basics of fitness training

* strength-training

* Cycling

* Running

* Running and Walking

* Push ups

* Stretching Exercises

* Strength-building Workouts

* Perform physical exercises.

Cases from Separate Sporting Fields

A number of international coaches and exercise experts have recommended that athletes follow a daily fitness program. George Payan is an expert trainer and is a regular trainer to sprinters. Payan asserts an internet training supply, http://www.coacheseducation.com, whereas he's elaborated on the everyday workouts by several kinds of athletes. A daily routine for 400-meter sprinters has been compiled by Payan. Payan's daily work outs start Monday and end on Monday. There are also periodic rest days.

Michael Phelps is a well-known swimmer who holds the record for the highest Olympic Gold, surpassing Mark Spitz. Phelps follows a strict daily regime. Phelps' unique characteristics can be distinguished from those of other men, however he still works hard six times a week. Jonathan P. Wade writes about his natural traits in Motley Health.

"Phelps, who is 6'4" tall, weighs in at 185lbs (84kg). His height is approximately 14 feet. He also has a 6ft 7in arm. His height gives him an advantage in the swimming pool. He has very short legs. In addition to having double-jointed knees and feet that can rotate 15 degrees faster than normal, his feet can also be turned fully so his flipper feet can function like flippers. These genetic traits allow him to kick the walls, then propel himself noodle as far as 10m.

Phelps' daily schedule includes six hours of 8 swimming or miles every day. He was usually at the pool by 6:30 am each day, twenty-six days a week, holiday included. Apart from his swimming, he does strength training. He spends approximately an hour per week strengthening his muscles, while only one hour daily on stretching his muscles. Phelps was known as "the individual Dolphin" because of the extent to which he can swim.

Olympic bumper plates can be crucial to any successful weight training program. There are many reasons why running a few dishes and a barbell is necessary. You might be training for a game or to increase your strength to weight ratio. Someone might be competing at a lifting competition. This could be cross-fit or strong-man. No matter your goal, you will need a barbell or a few plates. They are vital to your success in almost any aerobic workout.

People will often be taught to coach using only metal plates. These metallic plates cannot be tossed down like bare plates. To keep your weight down, don't lift any weights that are beyond your capabilities. You might not be getting the most out of your training if you don't lift weights which actually stimulate you. You need to ensure that you are training in a gym that has a wide range of food options, or to purchase a set yourself. While they're not very costly, make sure you stick to the highest quality plates. Do not buy cheap plates and then watch them fail in a few months. It is important to remember that weightlifting equipment can be an investment. You could possibly get some money back. In the unlikely event that you do not wish to sell the equipment, you could give it to your local gym or faculty or donate it to the children.

If you are smart and you need to own a few caliber Olympic bumper plates then you will require a barbell for those plates. When it comes to dishes and barbells, don't be cheap! The equipment can last a long time if properly maintained and calibrated. It is not something you want to do, like load a pub full of money and watch it become bent forever. A superb Bar-Bell could cost you around one hundred and fifty-five dollars. Spend three hundred to 500 dollars for a pub that could last you an entire lifetime. Pubs can be bought for hundreds of thousands of dollars. This makes it a good investment to have a pub that lasts a lifetime. If you stop lifting weights in ten years, you'll be able to promote a 400-dollar bar for around one hundred dollars.

This information is what you need to know. Go and purchase caliber Olympic Volt plates and a high-quality Bar Bell. We wish you all the best in your training, and we wish you every success.

"At every construction or house I have constructed, I have a plate with a bell"

These were the words of Ray "Thunder", an icon in professional wrestling, bodybuilding and entrepreneurship. (1)?In reality, dare I say that the Power of Thunder publication, which Ray Stern co-authored with Robert Wolff Ph.D., is the only source of information that can be trusted to give you the foundations of success in professional wrestling, bodybuilding, and entrepreneurship.

The circumstance of edifice creation was clarified. As a property agent and the leader of this business, Mr. Stern placed a significant barbell at the foundation of their homes and buildings. Stern explained, "I do it because I believe stimulation is a good thing. (two)

However, what about Bodybuilding? This could offer a blueprint for your lifetime success. How does your ability to achieve lasting, positive improvements to your body relate to the technical lessons of mind in setting goals.

Beyond the private Aspirations of success or definition of success body improvement may offer a microcosmic blueprint to bring dreams into reality. It does this with such determination that it can warn us about the potential dangers of shortcuts. For example, one of our long-term bodybuilding fans has never seen the novice musclebuilder that believes steroids are the answer to human progress. People might not see the long-term consequences of relying on these medications for their short-term gains. If we apply this observation to actual circumstances, it looks similar to Ray Stern's "Becoming great at every thing you do" principle. "Shortterm gain is consistent in calming long-term pain. Also, don't listen to anybody telling you otherwise." (3)

Aims: Your First Page on Your Success Blueprint

We need to have a clear internal representation of the things we want to be successful. A vague idea won't generate optimal outcomes. It is impossible to make an effective plan and stick to it if you are rambling through your day thinking things like "I want to get muscular" or "I wish to lose 1 fat". Our chances of achieving these goals increase if our goals are more specific.

This clinic can then applied to various situations. When you become skilled at setting specific goals for yourself, this skill will be instilled into your subconscious mind for effective recovery.

A Strong Strategy: The majority your Blue Print

Nothing can inspire you as much as a failure plan. It looks like this at the fitness center: A newcomer reads the instructions and decides to work on their knees every week. This person should do a balanced selection of exercises to obtain a number of 6-10 reps. It makes it possible for the person to increase their exercise, and even to train using "intensity", which is a fuzzy term. We must not forget to mention good form.

This film is a great movie. The first few weeks are fine. The only thing that will cause the progress plateau to be reached is an imperceptible, minor negative factor. Maybe the trainee's group amount is marginally higher than what they receive in rest - this variable isn't only linked to genetics. It also takes into account how stressed out she or he is and how often she sleeps. The following is possible: As a result of self-improvement, the trainee might unintentionally prepare for more difficult tasks. This could also be due to inadequate recuperation. It can become a frustrating way to lose motivation.

To solve this problem, you need to create a strategy that's effective. Not only highly effective. The power of a plan comes down to its flexibility and microfeedback. Flexibility means that your recovery and workout plan can be modified in small ways to make a significant difference. Micro-feedback can be described as a structured feedback that you can view from one work out to the next if you are on track. The feedback can serve as an instrument that allows for flexibility. If you don't react to the feedback, any work done is wasted. You can, provided you like to be rewarded for your efforts rather than doing moves.

What are the most important aspects of flexibility and Attention to details in establishing a solution that achieves our goals? Let us look at Ray Stern's Power of Thunder.

Visualization: A Homing Device

Arnold Schwarzenegger, the legendary Arnold Schwarzenegger, said that he loves his laps as giant hills onto his arms. Ray Stern wrote, "Think and think, consider your dreams and ambitions ..."(,"

Visualization can be used for body improvement if it is practiced and employed. You will find it easier and more effective the more you practice it. Your chances of achieving your goal rise dramatically when you visualize it and use positive emotions and enthusiasm to achieve it. All it takes is a few moments of silence every day. Your subconscious will begin to work on important points if you allow it to for a certain period of time. This is why this tool works as a homing system, directing you to the right thing.

You can imagine and even emotionallyize. You may be surprised at how little you know about your goal. It is gaining ten lbs of muscle. Then, stand in front of the bathroom scale and the mirror together with the beef slabs. When you lose twenty pounds of fat, visualize the slimmer version of yourself at the mirror. You might be promoted to a new job. In that case, you can visit your boss in her or his office. Let them know your progress and let you know how you feel.

The Supreme Success Principle Ground for Bodybuilding & Fitness

Bodybuilding and any other Form of Body Development are the best way to combine the world of your wants with the ability make these things happen. It's you, your whole body, and some equipment. You can get better results if you think outside the box. It is possible to reestablish the'success mentality.'

Chapter 4: Nutrition Is Crucial

A

Are you aware of how vital nutrition is for your body? You probably don't understand what you're actually feeding your body. Why do we eat? It's because you're likely hungry. However you might eat if bored, gloomy or tired. There are many reasons why people eat that way. A few of them may be physical like playing a game or emotional. Most likely, you do not consider why your body desires food. Not only does your body not need junk food, but it also requires healthy food that is great to nourish the whole body.

The nutrition you eat will provide energy for your whole body. Carbohydrates are essential for your body to have energy. Carbohydrates can be made from starch or sugar easily and are much more digestible than other foods. There are many ways to break down carbohydrate molecules into smaller pieces. All of these components are fructose-galactose-sugar. You might be surprised to learn that your body has its preferred form of energy. It's based on sugar. If your body takes in more carbs than you desire, it will start to store it.

There are many vitamins and minerals that can be obtained from what you eat. These are as vital for human health as carbs. Vitamins, antioxidants, and other compounds are known to aid the human body in compound responses. Some vitamins can help your body burn carbs, others aid you using vision, along with other vitamins that help with the functioning of your immune system.

So, nutrition is essential to ensure that your body has enough energy, nutrients, minerals and other structural components. Also, brightly colored vegetables can be beneficial to your health and help you stay healthy. You can find this with many vibrant fruits. Avocado seeds may contain anti-inflammatory properties, and apple skins might also have anti-oxidants that can help slow the aging process. You should have a range of colors to choose from, as this may help prevent and reduce certain issues with your wellbeing. All of these items can be found in your local community food shop.

Your body is your resource for nutrition. Nutrition is crucial for maintaining human anatomy health. The quality of your diet will impact how often you fall ill, how heavy and how healthy you become, as well as how long you can live. Three types of nutrition (carbs. protein. fats. and water) are a good example of the importance nutrition plays in our lives.

Carbohydrates can be a great source of energy. When consumed in the right amount, your body will experience optimal vitality. The surplus carbs will be converted into fats and stored in your system if they are not consumed in the correct volume. You start to feel heavier.

When concentrated fats are consumed in large volumes, they not only collect from the abdomen but also a compound in carbohydrates called cholesterol. Once they have accumulated in the bloodstream, they then float after congestion. You may experience internal bleeding.

Proteins are the building blocks of your human body's ability to repair and develop new muscles cells. The meal is best if you are looking to bulk up and build muscles. However, if you consume more fat than you desire, your system will make fats for storage. This is what you should know.

Water is vital too. Drink 8-10 glasses of pure water every day. Hydration is essential for your body to be able eliminate harmful wastes and maintain optimal digestion. Your body will be more susceptible to stroke, heart attacks, kidney disease, stomach disorders, and other potentially fatal maladies.

These situations will make it clear that nutrition is crucial to your well-being. Your well-being is the last thing you should compromise.

When you exercise and eat the right types of food, great nourishment can be easily achieved. To be nourished, you must have a healthy diet plan and avoid excessive eating. It is important to understand the nutritional requirements of your body if you want to have a healthy one. These foods refer to carbohydrates, protein and carbohydrates along with important minerals or vitamins.

A healthy lifestyle requires regular exercise and good nutrition. It is crucial to provide the body with the energy it needs. It's essential in maintaining healthy fats and strengthening the body's defenses. You can do any task well if you have a good weight. Regular exercise is crucial. You will be able to stay fit and active, which will certainly help with aging. It is important to enjoy the feeling that you are young, active, and strong. By doing this you can avoid serious diseases like overfatigue and other health issues.

It is difficult to comprehend the importance and effect nutrition has on general wellness. Neglecting to eat and malnutrition can both lead to bad health. In certain countries, a large number of people become sick due to insufficient food intake or nutrition. Obesity occurs when you eat more calories than your body needs. Obesity doesn't just cause aesthetic problems, but also contributes to higher blood pressure, higher blood glucose and back aches. Excessive fat, which can cause cholesterol, is a major factor in heart attacks and strokes. High salt intake can lead to elevated blood pressure and other serious health problems, such as heart attack or stroke. On the flipside, there are many states that disagree on how to tackle malnutrition in their area. Even though famine-related deaths can be quite common, they are not the norm. Some people may still have a diet lacking essential food nutrients, such vitamins, minerals and protein.

It is important to eat healthy food if you wish to live a healthy lifestyle. It is recommended to eat vitamin-enriched food in addition those with anti-oxidants. It is important to eat a balanced diet. Avoid sugary and sweet treats. Aim to consume lots of fluids. You need at least eight glasses water per day. This is important to keep your body hydrated.

A healthy balance is also essential when you choose the food that you eat. Eat healthy foods. Excellent nutrition is possible by choosing the right foods and portions. Keep in mind that your body requires all the nutrition elements of food to keep it healthy and strong. Maintain a healthy lifestyle to avoid any potential health risks. You will understand the importance and benefits of nutrition if your learn how to eat healthy foods, live in a healthy way of living. A healthy human body is the mirror of happy living.

Wikipedia describes nutrition as "A science that looks at the connection between diet, health, and nutrition." Bad nutrition may be responsible for some health issues, such as diseases. Let's examine the essentials of nutrition, and why it's so important for you.

How you feel could impact how you think, and how you respond to life on a daily basis. However, your beliefs could also affect how you feel. It is therefore important that you eat healthy foods that will help you live a happy and fulfilled life.

The worst thing that can happen to your nutrition is your creation of crap food. Proper nutrition is vital for a healthy body. Junkfood and takeout have lead to obesity and other health problems.

A lack of nutrition can lead to energy loss. This can also cause a lifestyle that involves sitting down and watching television, which can contribute to health problems. Many people will not wake up to be more productive. They often don't function properly, leading to obesity that can affect your health.

No doubt, changing your Diet is the first step in getting back control of your well-being. It is possible to feel healthier, lose weight, and improve your health. This could improve your self-esteem.

Chapter 5: Strength Or Hypertrophy?

A

All Game coaches may enjoy big. Many combative athletes, as well strong athletes, are keen to be big. Most trainers and athletes are not able to handle the challenge of training for strength and bulk simultaneously. The more an athlete pushes themselves, the more likely they are to reach a plateau by sticking with their existing routine. They can increase the quantity (a rise in places) or the seriousness (percentage just one rep max (maybe not sensed as muscle vexation), but it doesn't work. Volume training is great for increasing muscle mass and strength. However, it does not stimulate neural strength.

Neurological profits are usually used to increase muscle mass. Rep exercises can be more effective if they are performed correctly. Another issue that coaches and athletes face is that they must do high-intensity strength training to heal their nervous system (CNS).

The issue comes from the old saying that trainers can train hard or volume but not both.

T-Nation's Chad Waterbury suggests using a low (or higher) intensity bracket 75-85% to increase adaptability and decrease the rest periods (i.e. 10 sets of 3 with a minimum of 6 reps, and the remaining 60 seconds. Although I like this method, and it is not something I want to discourage, I believe there is another way. You can use the high strength bracket at 80 percent to 100 percent and you can increase your size AND strength by using sufficient volume.

The majority of participants and beginner athletes can achieve remarkable gains over the 60-70% power bracket. They are usually working towards 80 percent. The 80% rule means that your potency generally speaking will be stimulated beyond this percent. This typically demands a decline of places and a gain in rest periods. Most situations will see our method working beyond the 80% threshold.

Input Cluster Training

Cluster coaching isn't new. Actually, many Olympic weightlifters use this method without knowing it. Charles Poliquin, Christian Thibaudeau and Mike Mahler, just to name a few, were all able to devise this extremely effective way to lift this. Olympic weight lifters need to lose the weight in the bottom after each rep. That is often accompanied by a brief rest and then a second rep. Olympic weight lifters make the extremely heavy weight branch sport of weight lifting exceptionally muscular.

Cluster coaching allows an athlete (or trainee) to use intensity higher than the 80 percent threshold principle (generally, even higher 85-100percent). The coach uses sufficient volume to increase strength and size. Increased intensity and repetitions. This way of working is extremely demanding on the central nervous and should not be done by novices, freshmen, or sophomores in higher schools. It can be very effective, however, this should be limited to one elevator per movement band (flat pushing/pulling, vertical pushing/pulling, etc.). or just ONE exercise per body area. A second thing to remember is that you will need excellent spotters for this process. If you don't have at least one excellent spotter, you should not try this particular method. This is not just a way that is going to be kind for an athlete in case their spotter(s), need to take a break. Cluster training needs to be broken down, maybe not jumped into. I will show you a novel way to break cluster moving and teach more complex procedures. Coach Thibaudeau divides them in degrees. There is a degree inch that includes 3 techniques, and a degree 2 that contains 3 techniques. There is also a degree 3 which has 2 techniques. I'll be covering only degrees 1 and 2, while level 3 will follow shortly.

1,0

Coach Thibaudeau's elongated 5s technique is the first step to improve audience Training. The objective of the elongated5s process is to have an athlete do 10 repetitions using a load that is less than 5 repetitions. This really is a tremendous growth stimulant as there's an increase in strength, volume (85 percent x10 repetitions). So, this is an extended 5s set.

The athlete chooses 5 Repetitions (RM) that are most challenging and can do 5 repetitions before standing at the pub. After approximately 7-12 minutes of rest (recorded loudly by a spotter or exercise partner), the athlete un-racks his pub so that he can do another 2/3 repetitions. Once the 7-12 minute rest period is completed, the athlete can rack the pub for another 2-3 minutes. The last 23 repetitions will be accepted. The goal of the group is 10 repetitions. An athlete will typically only require two to 3 fractures to do this. The athlete takes a break for 3 minutes and then repeats it 3 times. This is a fantastic way to get started with audience training. Here's a short list...

Extended 5s method

Load- 80-85% from 1rm approximately 5 RM

Reps - 5 Reps with RM, 7-12 End. Reps 2-3 Reps 7-12 Pause. Reps 2-3 Reps

Sets- 3 5

Rush Intervals - 3-5 Minutes

Goal Target - 10 Repeats using a 5 RM

The classic bunch procedure is the next progression in audience Training. Charles Poliquin published a review of this technique in Modern Trends in Strength Training (2001).

Mike Mahler has also written articles on this particular technique, calling it Rest-Pause Training. It is a strong and efficient method, no matter its name. This technique is used to gain strength and hypertrophy in the type II-B muscles fibers. It's for people with potential power and force output. This procedure uses a greater intensity bracket than the elongated 5,s system. It usually uses 87-92percent to 1rm. It aims to reach intermitted repetitions for this specific load. So, a timeless bunch goes like this...

The athlete could pick from their 3-4 Repetitions max. Typically 35 places are used. Here's a short list...

Vintage Cluster Method

Load 85-92% of 1rm

Reps- 5 Total Reps, intermitted, Inch, pause, inch, pause, inch, pause, etc.,.

Sets- 3 5

Rush Intervals- 3-5 Minutes

Goal Target - Five Repetitions Using a 3-4 RM

The antagonist audience procedure is the Prior progress in degree 1. This is basically a variant of the traditional bunch procedure. With the exception that the athlete contrasts between opposing exercises using no remainder, (that is the pause accepted by the current conflicting exercise), this is an alternative to the traditional bunch procedure. The practice of a pair can still be used by reps and places, regardless of how it is done.

The athlete could pick their 3-4 repetitions maximum. After standing the pub, the athlete will complete 1 rep of bent-over barbell rows, 1 rep benchpress and 1 rep on this row. 35 positions are common. Here's a short list...

Antagonist Cluster Method

Load- 85-92% from 1rm

Reps - 5 Total Reps each antagonist Exercise. Rep Exercise inch. Rep Exercise Exercise two.

Sets- 3 5

Rush Intervals - 3-5 Minutes

Goal Target – 5 repetitions using a 3- 4 RM on two exercises

For People Who Need to Understand Antagonists, some examples include flat push and also push (seat & leg), vertical push and even vertical pull (shoulder pressing and palms upwards), four top notch dominant (squat & also decent morning), arms flake and extension of triceps.

Level 2

It doesn't matter if a Base of Audience Training was established in the previous degree, before moving on to the advanced techniques.

Mike Mentzer is the name of the moment Amount, which was developed at first. He was an accomplished bodybuilder. I was introduced to the Mentzer bunch process by Coach Thibaudeau's DVD on bunch training. Later, I read Weight Training The Mike Mentzer Way. This is a strong method that shouldn't be overlooked. This technique allows you to perform 4 to 5-5 repetitions while maintaining a 100-80percent commitment. At 90 100%

strength, the athlete can perform 23 singles and then lose 10 percent. A second 1 and 2 repetitions can then be done with this weight in timeless bunch fashion. Let's take an example:

The athlete chooses to do 98 percent of the 1RM. In addition, the athlete does inch rep. This is just one example...

Mentzer Cluster Method

Load - 90-98percent (1rm)

Reps- 4 5 Full Reps, intermitted, 1, 2 pause, 1, 2 pause, Inch, pause, lose weight 10 per cent, Inch Rep

Sets- 3 5

Rush Intervals - 3-5 Minutes

Goal Target - 4/5 Repeats with A1-3 RM

The Shed bunch is the 2nd type. This is a mixture of the Mentzer lot procedure and the traditional bunch system. A drop pair is, as most researchers know, a descending strategy for shedding weight. It can be performed after only a few repetitions. The shed group bunch maintains a high intensity (90 to 100percent) and loses weight by 5-10 pounds every single repetition. This time, the objective is to achieve 5 repetitions. For instance being...

The athlete will complete a rep with 98 to 100percent intensity. Then, the athlete stands at the pub while the spotters, or working partner, remove 5-10lbs from the pub. At the end of the seven-to-12-minute pause, the athlete stands again, Racks the bar, and spotters are able to lose 5-10 pounds further. Finally, the shed group bunch permits for high muscle strain due to the slow rate of repetitions and the rep has been completed in 100% maximum momentary force (i. All muscle fibers have been increasing being screened to increase the load. This list can be found here...

Fall Establish Cluster Method

Load 90 100% of 1rm

Reps- 5 Total Reps, intermitted, Inch, shed lower-weight 5 10 pounds, inch, shed lower-weight 5 10 pounds, inch, shed lower weight 5

10 pounds, inch Rep, shed weight 5 10 pounds, inch Rep, shed weightreduction

Sets- 3 5

Rush Intervals - 3-5 Minutes

Goal Target - 5 repetitions using a 1-3 RM

The highlighted bizarre audience procedure, the final step in degree 2, is known as the highlighted second progress. You will need a spotter to perform this technique. It may seem obvious, but I enjoy highlighting the weird parts of a workout (read Eccentric Training for Trainers article). This technique combines the timeless bunch approach with an emphasised eccentric part of the lifting. While the rep plot and group remain close to the timeless bunch, however, during the bizarre or decreasing portion of the practice, your working partner will push you back on the pub. It requires an exceptionally skilled spotter! They should use just enough immunity for the athlete to lower the bar! If the pub is falling like bricks, it isn't helping them. Here's an excellent illustration.

The athlete could pick 3-4 repetitions maximum. In order to do inch reps with all their training partners, pressure is applied to the pub at the diminishing%. Usually, 35 places are utilized.

There will always be disagreements over effective weight training program design. My entire career as an instructor has been a mix of various hypertrophy and power training methods. The fact that these apps encourage what I perceived to be totally antagonistic coaching methods was something that always interested me. One pro will say that only large-volume training is ideal for muscle building, while another pro will agree that training at a lower level and with higher intensity is important. You would spend more time looking at the complicated variations of other patterns than you would training. This can also be called "analysis paralysis".

What was evident was that, despite contradictory information being presented, the best applications usually share common elements or fundamentals. It will not be a matter of emphasizing individual notions but instead, it will examine the larger picture: the principles. This guide's goal is to provide the best training fundamentals in a simple, clear way. These are the basic principles that will benefit you when you design your next app. This really is what "Really Works" when it concerns instruction for strength or size.

Inch. Progressive Overload:

Here's the Standard and most essential axiom. While they adapt to stress, muscle grows stronger and larger. This is why you need to overload your muscles every week by lifting slightly less weight, using more force, or doing more repetitions of the exact weight loss. This is why it is essential to record your progress as well as your training goals.

2. You can use chemical-free weight exercises

Basic, large pulling, pushing, motions such as this dead lift and lunge, squat and lunge variations, power wash overhead press chest press row, pullup, and power washing require bigger exercises, greater muscle bands, higher immunity, and greater Neuro Muscular Activation (NMA). These movements are more demanding than isolation moves. The NMA will increase the longer you practice the exercise and the farther you go. The reason why a large recoil dip is more efficient than other media is that pullups are more complex than pullbacks. These exercises are more effective than other methods, allowing for greater size and intensity gains over a shorter period of time. Additionally, they stimulate the creation high levels of human growthhormones within the human system. De-stabilized training (free weights, machines) might allow you to engage smaller muscles.

3. Ground-based Exercises are a good idea.

This idea can be used in conjunction with all the Principles. You can coach at a standing position, or a ground-based position that is in place of lying or sitting. This alone will make the exercise easier and more functional. Comparing the padded overhead media to standing military media or bent-over dumbbell racks to compare, you can see how they are much more functional. You'll also notice a greater engagement of your heart muscles with earth-centered exercises.

4. Teach your CORE:

Some people identify their heart as their Abdominals. But I also examine their "heart", which is the whole of the waist. It is worth considering that you need to incorporate exercises to target these main areas. For a stronger workout and protection against injury, I recommend starting your exercise with some heart isometrics. The board, the bridge's medial side, and the rear expansion would be the principles. I finish each piece with a different isotonic exercise.

If you are doing large, multi-joint exercises like I mentioned, your heart muscles may be strained throughout the rest of the work out. Your entire waist will be involved when you use functional, freeweight and ground-based chemical motions. Because of the potential for reducing the heart stabilizers' engagement, I strongly discourage the use of straps, wraps, and straps in your daily routine. These accessories are best used to increase lift efforts and rivalry, except where otherwise advised.

5. Train using Balance:

I have written many articles on the subject of 'balance'. They include: Assessing training and rest, training different energy systems to balance; finding balance in one's own life. It's an important subject and shouldn't be overlooked. Let's look at the next facets to equilibrium.

O Unilateral (single leg, arm) and firmness training

Include some exercises that help one focus on one leg or stabilize one-arm burdens. These include single-arm presses, measure ups, and workouts. Working with unusual items, such as sandbags and kegs, can also increase your need for stabilizers. It can also cause a new strain on the human body. These kinds of moves increase the potency one's poorer positive and also improve your proprioceptive ability.

O Balance exactly how much training is required to attain (aswell as the potential of) agonist or antagonist (conflicting?) muscle bands:

This is a crucial principle in order to increase strength, size, NMA, and prevent harms. Ostensibly, this means that you must balance the workload between your driving and pulling movements. These antagonist muscles are responsible for eccentrically stabilizing the joint. This will affect the drive and rate you can generate at a media, or throw. If you can't control deceleration then you won't be able accelerate to your full potential.

A Place to establish an antagonist muscle between two places has been shown to speed up recovery. You can call these Pushpull Supersets. These include super-setting rows and trunk presses or Pull Ups. It has been demonstrated to preserve potency, as well as spark hypertrophy.

O Function in Your own Muscular Imbalances

Muscle strain is frequently caused by joint pain or weakness. This is where isolation exercises come in. To help your weak connections, you will need to train them until they are able to be included in a movement design. Otherwise, your muscles may not last long enough to compensate for the loss. Anterior deltoids are the most prominent cases of poor connections. They also include the outside rotator band, anterior deltoids. Lower trapezius. Glute medius. Vasus medialus. And often, some heart muscle.

To sum it all, it's a waste to do a whole workout with isolation exercises for smaller muscular groups (unless you're in a rehab program / pre-hab). One hour of workout that is simply "arms", for example, will not be noticed. Each workout should excite the vast majority, with exercises that require fewer. Train moves, not muscles.

"Functional training" (incorporated exercise), is only able to fortify compensatory patterns when the weak connections haven't been identified.

-- Greg Roskopf, MA, creator Muscle Activation Methods

6. Conduct Strong-man Implement Training

Strong Man odd and training thing. Lifting is great for improving a trainee's general physical readiness (GPP) as well as stimulating new neural muscle recruit routines. Exercises like sleddraggingfarmers walk or keg press, thick pub lifts or sandbag conveys can increase the use of muscles that are not easily contested by a barbell. It also provides a lot of stimulation for your own heart muscles and small joint stabilizers.

It is possible to combine strong man training with many of the axioms mentioned above (#2,3,4& 5). This includes functional, chemical and ground-based movements that increase heart strength and balance. Strong man training is a fun and effective way to increase your workout efficiency. It can be easily integrated into your training program. Try it.

7. Training in Explosiveness and Containment Rate:

Powerful muscles are essential to maximize your potential power. Speed training is a great way to build more power. (Power equals Force-X Rate). Plyometric, sprint, and Olympic Weightlifting exercises are all powerful. This helps prepare your body for the sudden changes in your lifestyle and competition. A great strength trainer once said "Life's Ballistic." Get ready to do it.

8. Use the Procedure of Periodization

It is possible to reap the long-term benefits of app periodicization if you follow a few steps. A periodization strategy is an exercise plan that incorporates suggested workout times, strength, volume, and workout choice. Terminal periodization is the preferred Western technique. It divides different aspects into different phases. But, it has many limitations. Conjugated or short-term periodization can be very effective, but it is more time-consuming. In contrast, conjugated periodization allows you to train many aspects of strength, such as maximum strength and vibrant intensity, with the same weekly schedule. Louie Simmons at Westside Barbell Club applied this process. There are other options, including pendulum-training, but I won't belaboring on this. However, I strongly recommend you to consider periodization and adopt a method that meets your needs.

9. Version:

Many people are aware that instruction load must be increased. However, a few individuals seem to recognize that the stimulation for training should also be varied periodically to keep the body and nervous systems stimulated to adapt.

Your progress will decrease if you keep doing the exact same workouts, using the exact exact same sequences of exercises and the exact same set and reps. It is important to constantly change the exercises to challenge your body and make it adapt to new stresses. Contain unique rep ranges (i.e. You should have a unique rep range (e.g., decreased repetitions for maximum strength and rate training, medium repetition range for hypertrophy or high repetitions for endurance), and you should also change your primary exercises every 36 week. This can be adapted by a well-designed periodization system such as the westside.

10. Give yourself enough time:

Muscles are developed while you're at rest. Although immunity is what stimulates growth, it's also how you sleep, eat, and rest that allows hypertrophy. Most people are busy and need 6 to 8 hours of quality sleeping each night. The amount depends on how much they train, eat, sleep, and what their stress levels are.

In order to maximize the amount of rest during the workout, heavy, maximum-effort lifting sets (i.e. : 2 to 4, and less between sets to achieve a slower rate or endurance training (i.e. The duration of the session is 60-90 minutes. The greater the group's severity, the more time between parts is required. Your ability to rest longer could cause your lactic acids levels to drop, which can limit your operations on the next group.

It is also a good idea to increase the length of your workout. It's possible for you to work out your strength between 30 and 60 minutes. This will give you a boost of growth hormones at the end. This will improve your healing. Training for too long could result in a drop of your natural anabolic degree and impede your restoration. You may feel tired and weak.

Hypertrophy occurs when Muscles contract and produce more force. This is especially true for athletes who need to have a large muscle mass. Strength training is an ideal way to increase muscular hypertrophy. Weight training may be difficult or it could be done just right to achieve your goals.

Let us first examine the results at the cellular level of this training before I explain Ideal Training to market hypertrophy and endurance. Also, protein elements are created when muscles contract. The most important protein components are the mysosin or actin filaments. They make slip cross bridges, bridges that induce. A muscle has 1000s such filaments. This makes it difficult to create a lot of power and force.

Your body will have to adjust to increased muscle stress during immunity training. This raises both myosin- and actin-fibrill count. Increased myosin, actin filaments and sarcomeres levels in muscle tissues leads to greater amounts of these sarcomeres. While the size of muscle fibers won't increase, it is not possible to stop them from growing. These gains can take some time before you notice them. The muscle fibers will grow slowly and, most importantly, it will take seven weeks for the significant gap to appear.

Ok, now you understand the fundamental Cellular quantity responses. What is the best training that increases substantial muscle hypertrophy and strength?

Repeated lifting of heavy weights is required to train muscles. It is important to copy, but how much weight is needed to make the practice profitable?

Many people discuss the importance of quantity training. Imagine that you do three sets of 8-10 reps. That would give you about half a dozen repetitions. This is a fantastic way to track progress over weeks and months. The only thing you have to do is decide how much weight your body takes. Therefore, a pair might contain ten repetitions.

For example, if you decide to build three places every day but you are also aware that it is a difficult task to do ten repetitions for thirty kilograms, you won't be able lift that weight. Keep your repetitions and sets steady by lifting lighter weights. Do your homework to ensure your body has access to water and proteins. Otherwise, you will not be able promote strength.

For example, hemadrol is a protein-nutritional supplement. If you don't expect nutritional supplements that Aren't legal, then the product like hemadrol will be best for you. It's legal as well as offering a money-back warranty.

Chapter 6: What Is Your Goal

You have heard it millions of times. What is your goal. I'm referring to your goal and body weight for this book. Most will say, "I want the most weight I can lift." However, they are often unaware that your weight affects the amount of weight you can lift. Weigh classes wouldn't be needed if that were the case. This seems obvious, but I want to stress that it will still apply if you adopt or transition to a more vegetable-based diet.

Strength is very personal. For a 60kg lifter, 225lbs is not a lot. However, it is dependent on the bodyweight of the lifter. What is the definition of strong? Do you know what is strong?

These statements are not new to you.

"Vegans are small and weak because they don't get enough nutrition."

"I once tried veganism and ended up losing my strength."

I had the former mentality before I tried vegan. However, after my failed attempts, the latter drove me to return to animal products. Here's an example of what a failed vegan might experience.

The people have either come across a convincing documentary on animal rights (can you suggest Earthlings)? Or they have seen convincing arguments for eating more plant-based foods. They're ready to transition and become fully vegan. They may go full speed ahead and begin a vegan diet that could be completely different to what they have used to. Even if they aren't tracking their calories it is possible that they have a normal routine diet that they consider to be healthy. Their body will adapt to what they see before it takes months, if not years to adjust to their specific diet and exercise level. When they go vegan completely, or even partially, they accidentally change their total calories and/or their macronutrients ratio. Their individual macronutrient mix is how many calories they have been able to get from carbohydrates, protein, fat, and other nutrients.

A person's body type can be greatly affected by their calorie intake and macronutrient intake. A male weighing in at 210 lbs could have consumed around 3000 calories. These calories contained 60% Carbs (25%) Protein and 15% Fat. The person could consume 2400 calories from a plant-based diet if he or she switches to 75% Carbs. They also get 10% protein and 15% Fat. One small shift over a few months can lead to significant changes in the male. Perhaps he notices his strength decrease and loses weight. This could not happen if the person knew how many calories he had and what percent of each macronutrient.

Sources indicate that the amount of calories and the percentage of macronutrients affect the strength and weight of the body.

This addresses what is probably the biggest concern for strength athletes regarding plant-based nutrition. If you're not paying attention, the answer is usually yes. I have yet to meet anyone who has not lost weight after adopting a plant-based lifestyle. These two words make it more accurate, but I forgot to include them. The words are "Whole Foods." Do you know anyone, even hypothetically, who could be considered overweight if they only consumed fruits and veggies that were not high in fat? Most fruits and vegetables have low levels of fat and high amounts of carbohydrates. Whole food plant-based eating will result in a lower calorie intake, fewer processed foods, higher fiber intake, and more satisfaction. It will also help to reduce psychological cravings related to processed foods. You may already see where I am heading with this.

"Ultimately, macronutrient absorption and calories are what will determine your relative success or failure when you adopt a plant-based lifestyle.

I don't want to get into IIFYM, but I do believe it works. This rule has one notable exception, which I and others have found to be true. If an active person consumes normal calories but follows a high carb, low fat diet, it seems that this will cause a slight weight loss.

"Dr. John McDougall has discovered, over the course of his lifelong research, that eating a starch-based diet high carbohydrate, low fat, and low protein could have many positive health effects.

He claims that the abundance of carbohydrates can be stored as energy, used to make body heat, or stored as energy. This might be the best way to maintain a healthy weight. For the strength athletes who don't desire to see a dramatic weight loss, they may actually want to gain weight.

Although diet is essential for strength athletes, the most important thing is how they feel about themselves (strong or poor) and their body type. You may notice an increase or decrease of weight by changing your diet to vegan, or making other semi-radical diet changes. Weight loss can lead to a person becoming weaker or getting heavier. I don't want to see lifters abandon the baby with a bad approach.

It is crucial to pay close attention calories depending on what body type you have. A person who is lean with a high metabolic speed may have difficulty gaining weight. High carbohydrate intake is recommended for vegan barbell players. This provides adequate carbs for barbell training. Different bodies react differently to different vegan diets. For instance, people with heavy body weight have difficulty losing weight. Carbohydrate rich diets can cause weight gain. These vegan barbell trainers with carb intolerance need to eat a healthy diet rich in protein and fat, which includes fruits and vegetables.

Chapter 7: Choose Your Body Type

This chapter title might confuse you. I do not claim to have the ability to alter your genes. Nor am I trying to minimize the work involved in changing one's body. Individuals' current and/or genetic bodyweight depend on many factors such as age, gender, exercise level, training history, nutrition, and other factors.

This book is about how adopting a vegan lifestyle or transitioning to one can affect your current weight and progress. A few situations might arise if you follow a vegan diet.

You will lose weight.

You will gain weight.

You'll maintain your weight.

Consider whether you're losing or gaining muscle/fat.

The question of what your ideal bodyweight is can be very difficult and confusing. As I mentioned in the previous chapter high carb low fat vegans experts often explain that following this diet will "normalize" your bodyweight. Generally, I find that the weight mentioned is close to one's ideal Body Mass Index.

There are many people who have concerns about the body Mass Index. I am one of them. It is hard to pinpoint the "ideal" weight without taking into consideration bone density, activity level, and mass. However, I have found that the suggested BMI range for high carbohydrate low fat vegans is quite close in numbers. Although I don't want to be judgmental about you if your passion is lifting heavy items and carrying around some extra weight, I will suggest alternatives. You should be aware that going vegan and not going over the "obese" line of BMI may not be the best choice for your body. Last but not least, there is a huge difference between Nutrition for Health (or Sports Nutrition) and Nutrition for Strength Nutrition.

Katherine Beals and others like her have found one constant, which is different from other diets. The LFPBD (whole food plant-based diet) will help you lose weight. This can be due to many factors, but especially because plant foods are typically low in fat, low protein, and high carbohydrate. It is easy to notice the slimming of these doctors and their patients. This may not be for you if strength athletes are your goal. This is why I emphasize the importance of the question: What is your goal and what is your ideal weight? For simplicity, I have listed four basic body types. These can be adjusted depending on what your diet is.

Because of the complexity of our anatomy, physiology and biology, I apologize for dividing different body types into 4 groups. Did I mention this book was meant to be easy? Important note: If you have a natural tendency to be a certain height or weight, it's best to not push the limits of your mother nature. If you're 5'2" it is likely that you don't want to try for the super heavyweight category.

The relationship between diet and body type is very strong. Here are some facts about the relationship between body types and diet

People with a thin and fragile body need to consume a lot of calories to gain weight. Because of their high carbohydrate tolerance and fast metabolism, they burn calories quickly. These people may wish to increase their size by consuming more fat and protein.

A person with little to moderate weight has a middle body structure. A mixed diet with balanced carbohydrate (protein, fat, and carbohydrate) is a good option for little overweight people.

People with large body fat and an inefficient metabolism rate are more likely to gain weight than people who are overweight. An athlete might find that a low-fat high-carb vegan diet is the perfect way to lose weight. They should do this if they wish to lose their weight.

Here is a breakdown for different body types, and arbitrary bodyweights.

Men

Featherweight (123lb-152lbs)

Light Heavyweight (185lbs-207lbs)

Heavyweight(207lbs-231lbs)

Super Heavyweight (231-31 lbs - 300 lbs).

Women

Strawweights (up to 115lb

Bantamweight (115-135lbs).

Women's Light Heavyweight (135lbs-170lbs).

Women's Heavyweight (170lbs - 200lbs)

Are you wondering why I chose these numbers? These numbers represent a combination of Mixed Martial Arts and Olympic Lifting weight classes.

Once you have determined your ideal or desired weight, the next chapter will explain the different macronutrients that could support it.

Chapter 8: Macronutrient Breakdown According To Body Types And Goals

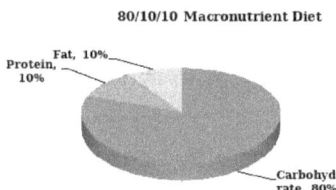

80/10/10 Macronutrient Diet

Calories, which are the primary indicator of one's dietary intake to maintain or alter body structure, are everything. Even though they have a lot of calories, vegans can still lose weight with certain plant-based approaches. I discovered this while following Dr. Doug Graham's 80/10/10 diet (80% Carbs, 10% Protein, 10% Fat), as suggested by T. Collin Campbell and Dr. John McDougall. It dawned on me that Dr. McDougall's old quote, "The Fat You Eat is the Fat You Wear" was true.

This table is based on my personal experience, the sources of professional vegan strength-athletes, and the literature. It provides an overview of approximate macronutrients breakdown for each weight category, along with their diet.

A standard table of macronutrient breakdown based upon generic body types

Is it possible to guess which vegan would adopt the following categories of body weights and macronutrient breaks? Experts in diet and professional trainers have shown me that a casual American weightlifter will most likely shift to one of the two options. Either they mimic their old diet and eat a greater portion of the 40/30/30/30 or they choose to eat 80/10/10. This is a 180-degree change from what their body used to.

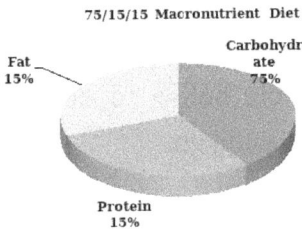

75/15/15 Macronutrient Diet

Fat 15%

Carbohydrate 75%

Protein 15%

Featherweight / Strawweight Macronutrient: 80/10/10

Description: This is not surprising for vegans and other non-vegans. Eating whole fruits, vegetables, and vegetables won't cause weight gain. This is why Dr. Neal Barnard, Dr. Douglas Graham, T. Collin Campbell, and Dr. John McDougall all highly recommend them. If you are not familiar with these people, I recommend looking them up. Because of their gender, women might also be in this category.

But don't let it stop you from training with the barbell. It is possible to increase your strength and maintain it in this weight group. A 80/10/10 macronutrient-based diet that builds strength at higher weights can result in a decrease in weight. This weight loss will result in a decrease in the weight you can lift. Be aware that strength is directly related to body size. Simply refer to the table below to determine where your numbers should go.

Light Heavyweight: 70/15/15

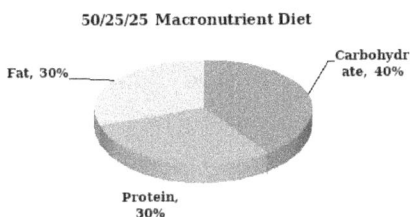

Fat, 30%
Carbohydrate, 40%
Protein, 30%

Description: It will become apparent that as the fat and protein percentage increases, the carbohydrate intake slightly decreases. This slight change in the carbohydrate intake over the course of time can help athletes be more productive in the weightroom. You'll be amazed at the results of this particular diet when you do barbell training. A 70/15/15 macronutrient diet can be used to strengthen the body. This ratio is best for a lean and muscular look.

Heavyweight: 50/25/25

Description: For this body type, increasing the proportion of fat and proteins is the best way to get it. Vegan barbell athletes need to ensure that they eat enough protein. For any strengthening exercise, increasing your protein intake can help increase muscle development. As a vegan, it's natural to worry that a plant-based diet could deprive your body protein, which is essential for bodybuilding. Some of the best sources for protein are foods such as tofu, soy, legumes, beans and other beans. Vegan protein rich food is a good source for protein and fiber. The 50/25/25 macronutrient regimen is beneficial for vegan athletes looking to achieve a more muscular physique with moderately low body weight.

Super Heavyweight (40/30/30)

40/30/30 Macronutrient Diet

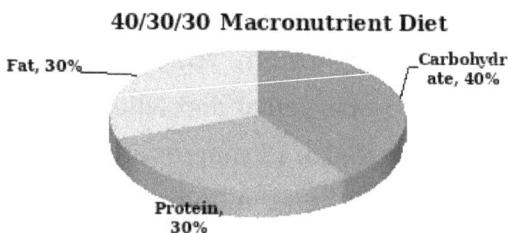

Fat, 30%

Carbohydrate, 40%

Protein, 30%

Description: This body type prefers a 40/40/20 micronutrient diet. This is the best option if your goal is MASS. While it may not be good for your overall health, it is better for your heart. The amount of fat, protein and carbohydrates that you consume will increase dramatically when you include carbohydrate. A sound training program will ensure that you get the fat increase and the protein. You will notice an increase of weight lifting when you have this extra weight stored. The super heavyweight vegan will have the ability to lift weights by training with vegan barbells. Many will not believe that such a Mass Monster is vegan.

Diet: All of the above-mentioned food with the inclusion of faux meats and vegan-processed food.

Chapter 9: Training Goals For Each Body Type

Training numbers: Below is a table that shows approximate ranges, averages, and the results of different barbell exercises. There are two possible options: you can fall within the range of your weight or go beyond these thresholds. It's safe to say that athletes who are middle-weight or lower in these ranges, but still want to lift weights within their range, will need additional training. This is acceptable, especially if your training has been for less than one to three years. It is also obvious that your Olympic lifts training will not be as effective as if only you are doing powerlifts.

It is strongly advised that vegan strength athletes maintain high standards. This should not be an issue for anyone who follows a plant-based diet.

Chapter 10: Shopping List Based Upon Goals

Weight Class	Calorie Range	Snatch Range	Clean and Jerk Range	Squat	Bench	Deadlift
123lbs-152lbs (69kg-77kg)	2100—2500	94lbs-209lbs	88lbs-242lbs	300lbs—365lbs	195lbs—225lbs	315lbs—405lbs
185lbs-207lbs (85kg-94kg)	2500—2700	209lbs-220lbs	242lbs—330lbs	405lbs—450lbs	265lbs—300lbs	425lbs—470lbs
207lbs-231lbs (94kg—>105kg)	2700—3000	209lbs—264lbs	242lbs—319lbs	405lbs—>475lb	265lbs—>375lbs	425lbs—>500lbs
231-300lb 105kg-136kg	3000-4000	264-345lbs	319->400lbs	475lb—515lbs	375lbs—>405lbs	500lbs—600lbs

It is essential that this shopping list be simple. This list isn't meant to be exhaustive. There are many whole and processed foods that can be purchased. Also, you may notice a rising number of processed foods. This isn't to say that it shouldn't be done! I think we all can agree that nuts and avocados make healthier choices than refined oil. These ingredients are based on the amount of macronutrients that have been broken down. The list can include a wide range of ingredients that can be selected based upon one's body type.

Shopping list

Chapter 11: Faq (More Information Will Be Added Soon).

Q. Q.

A. Vegans will not experience a loss of strength at first. All the essential nutrients are available to the body through a vegan diet. Even if I didn't make the case, training and caloric consumption will directly impact strength.

Q. Q. Are vegan protein products as effective as

80/10/10	75/15/15	50/25/25	40/30/30
Apples	Previous Column +	Previous Columns +	Previous Columns +
Apricots	1-2oz Nuts/Seeds	>2oz Nuts/Seeds	Crackers
Bananas	Beans (Dried or	Avocados	Refined Oil
Beets	Canned)	Bread	Vegan Meat
Bell Peppers	Grains (Whole)	Cheese Substitute	Substitutes
Berries	Legumes	(Dairy)	
Broth (Vegetable)	Milk Substitute (Soy	Olives	
Cantaloupe	or Nut)	Protein Powder	
Carrots	Pasta	(Vegan)	
Celery		Nut Butters	
Cereal		Tomato Sauce	
Cherries		Tofu	
Corn		Tempei	
Dates		Seitan	
Eggplant		Quinoa	
Grapes			
Lettuce			
Mangos			
Mushrooms			
Nectarines			
Onions			
Pineapple			
Potatoes			
Prunes			
Rice			
Spinach			
Strawberries			
Tomatoes			
Watermelon			
Tapioca			
Maple syrup			

whey?

A. Yes, vegan protein supplements are just as effective and as efficient as whey proteins. Even better! The majority of vegan proteins come from plant sources (mostly organic), which contain all the amino acids and have naturally occurring vitamins, minerals, fiber, and vitamins. You are definitely losing more than you gain. Sunwarrior's, Plant Fusion's, and Garden of Life are my top recommendations.

Q. Q.

A. Your diet is not compromised by avoiding animal products. While some may be concerned about vitamin B12, it is an essential component of the diet for meat eaters. No matter what type of diet you follow, it is a good idea that you take a B12 vitamin supplement. If you are eating from a variety plant sources, a vegan diet provides all the necessary nutrients for your body. Vegetarian diets also contain fiber, vitamin B, and other nutrients that can't be found in animal products.

Q. Q.

		80/10/10	75/15/15
Breakfast	Day 1	1 glass of Pineapple Grape Fruit Delight 1 large bowl of Blue and Red Fruit Salad	1 glass of sunrise delight juice 2 slices of whole wheat bread Scrambled tofu with fresh veggies
	Day 2	1 large bowl of Fresh Fruit Treat Green Specks Watermelon Juice	Superfood breakfast 1 glass of fresh, tender coconut water
	Day 3	Orange Hue Assorted Fruit Mix	1 bowl of Creamy Fruit Delight Banana Date Smoothie
Lunch	Day 1	1 large bowl of Creamy Squash Salad Raw Mango Vegetable Mix 1 cup steamed rice	1 bowl of Healthy Salad 1 cup of brown rice Spicy Lentil Vegetable Curry
	Day 2	Hot and Sweet Burritos 2 slices of brown bread	Pasta in Rich Tomato Gravy
	Day 3	Tapioca Fruit Surprise 2 slices of fruit bread with maple syrup	Aromatic Vegetable Rice
Dinner	Day 1	Mixed Vegetable Rice Soup	Beet and Carrot Noodles with Spicy Vegetables
	Day 2	Gingery Beet Carrot Soup Lemony Steamed Vegetables	Cinnamon Vegetable Soup 2 slices of French bread Toast
	Day 3	1 cup steamed brown rice Mashed Seasoned Potatoes Tangy salad	Red Pasta With Tofu and Vegetables

A. A. Don't believe any negative reviews about soy. I haven't experienced any side effects from soy and I haven't been without it for more than 2 days. You can always stop eating it if it causes you discomfort. There are many options.

Q. Q.

A. Vegan Bodybuilding & Slapping by Robert Cheeke. Derek Tresize presents The Vegan Muscle and Fitness Guide. Veganbodybuilding.com. 30Bananasaday.com Adaptt.org.

Q. Q.

It is still a matter of debate whether raw or cooked vegans are the best. Ethical vegans won't mind if your lifestyle includes chips and french fries. Plant-based health advocates might respond by saying, "You could as well just eat animal products."

Surprisingly, consuming vegetables and plants in their raw form makes complete sense. All the logic that humans are the only living creature in the food chain who prepare their food makes it seem very reasonable. T. Collin Campbell (Dr. John McDougall), and Caldwell Esselstyn (Dr. Caldwell Esselstyn) are all expert cooks who have a strong track record in improving health using cooked (minimally processed). Which one is better? Most people will not be able to decide which one is the best until they see enough raw and cooked vegans over 110 years of age.

		50/25/25	40/30/30
Breakfast	**Day 1**	Creamy and Nutty Fruit Salad 2 slices of banana bread	1 glass of Detoxifying Juice Coconut Stuffed Pancakes
	Day 2	Mung Beans and Coconut Salad	Banana Almond Smoothie 2 slices of brown bread with peanut butter
	Day 3	Quinoa Coconut Milk Porridge	Quinoa Oatmeal with Toasted Almonds
Lunch	**Day 1**	Tofu and Vegetables with Rice Noodles	Chili Tofu Noodles
	Day 2	1 bowl of Vegan Sweet Potato Avocado Cream Salad	Red Kidney Beans Curry with Indian Bread
	Day 3	Carrot Beetroot Fry with Shredded Coconut 2 slices of flat Indian Bread Protein Punch	Quinoa Tomato Mint Salad 1 slice of brown bread
Dinner	**Day 1**	Beet and Carrot Noodles with Mashed Black Bean	Hot and Sweet Quinoa Bowl
	Day 2	Tempered Quinoa With Vegetables	Asparagus and Red Quinoa Salad
	Day 3	Vegetables and Tofu with Mashed Kidney Bean	Plaintain and Tofu in Coconut Gravy

Raw fruits and veggies can sometimes be more nutritious than cooked ones, as some of the delicate vitamins are greatly destroyed during cooking.

For instance, raw tomatoes contain a lot more vitamin C than cooked tomatoes. The ease of digestion is ensured by using cooked cauliflowers. You can use either raw or cooked ingredients to achieve the following ratios. For athletes who prefer an all-raw diet, you can remove the * items.

Chapter 12: Food Planning And Recipes

FOOD PLANNING

Recipes

Smoothies and Juices

Fruit Salads

Vegetable Salads

Breakfast

Main Course Lunch/Dinner

Smoothies and juices

Green Specks Watermelon Juice

Ingredients

2 cups Cubed watermelon cubes

Fresh basil leaves – Fistful

1/2 cup crushed ice

Method

Mix watermelon cubes in a blender with crushed ice. Mix basil leaves in a blender and blend until you get green specks.

* Top with fresh basil leaves and serve in tall glasses

Sunrise Delight

Ingredients

1/3 cup of cooked tapioca

1/2 cup orange slices

Pineapple slices 1/2 cup

1/2 cup crushed Ice

Honey 1 teaspoon

Method

Blend the pineapple and orange slices together in a blender. Mix honey with orange slices.

* Place the cooked tapioca in a large glass.

Serve with crushed ginger

Pineapple Grape Fruit Delight

Pineapple chunks : 1 cup

Red grapefruit : 1

1 tsp.

Some crushed ice

Method

* Blend grapefruit, pineapple chunks, and grated Ginger in a juicer

* Season with black sea salt, and serve the pineapple grapefruit delight in tall glasses filled with crushed ice

Detoxifying juice

Ingredients

Spinach : 2 cups packed

Parsley - 1/4 cup

Mint leaves : 1/4 cup

Lemon juice : 1 TSP

1 tsp.

Method

* Wash all green leaves well under running water. Blend them together in a juicer

* Combine lemon juice with black salt.

Banana Date Smoothie
Ingredients

1 cup. Peeled, sliced and chopped ripe bananas

Pitted dates : 1/2 cup

1/2 cup of green cardamom pulverize

Maple syrup 1/2 cup

Method

Blend all ingredients in a bowl and then serve in a tall glass with basil leaves.

Orange Hues
Ingredients

Peeled and chopped carrot - 1/2 cup

Ripe grapefruit slices : 1/3 cup

Cubed ripe papaya : 1/2 cup

Crushed Ice - 1/2 Cup

Method

Mix all ingredients and pour into a large glass. Garnish with apple slices

Banana Almond Smoothie

Ingredients

Half cup of sliced ripe banana

Soaked almonds – 5-6

Soy milk - 1 cup

1/2 tsp. green cardamom powder

1/2 cup crushed ice

Crushed cashew nuts 2 tbsp

Method

* Combine all ingredients in a juicer. Blend well. Mix all ingredients in a blender until smooth. Serve in a glass.

Creamy, nutty fruit salad

Ingredients

1/2 cup chopped ripe banana

Cubed pineapple : 1/2 cup

Blackberries - 1/4 cup

Mashed ripe avocado : 1 cup

Crushed almonds 1 tbsp

1 tbsp.

Vanilla essence : 1 tsp.

Maple syrup: 1 Tbsp.

Method

* Place all ingredients in a bowl. Chill.

Fruit Salads

Coconut Salad and Mung Beans

Ingredients

Yellow mung beans : 3/4 cup

Grated coconut - 1/2 cup

Sliced bananas: 1

Crushed cashewnuts : 1 Tbsp

Soaked raisins : 2 tbsp.

1/4 cup grated jaggery

Method

* Pour water over mung beans to soak them overnight

* Toss the soaked mung Beans in a salad bowl.

Creamy Fruit Delight

Ingredients

Sweet corn - 1 Cup

Peeled and cubed pineapples - 1/2 cup

Cherries: 1/4 cup

Peeled and cubed ripe mangoes - 1/2 cup

Maple syrup: 2 Tbsp.

Method

To cook the sweet corn, microwave it for a couple of minutes. Blend the half-cup of sweet corn to make a smooth paste in a blender. Combine the remaining corn with water to make a coarse paste.

* Add the cherries, mangoes and pineapple pieces to a large bowl. Use a spatula and gently mix the prepared corn mixture over the fruits.

* Refrigerate for few minutes. Make creamy fruit delights and serve chilled with maple syrup.

Fresh Fruit Treat

Ingredients

1/4 cup cubed apple -

Grapes: 1/4 cup

1/4 cup cubed pineapples

Sliced peaches - 1/4 cup

Sliced bananas: 1/2 cup

Vanilla essence : 1 tsp.

Water: 1/4 cup

Fresh basil leaves : 4 - 5

Maple syrup: 2 Tbsp.

Method

* Add the chopped bananas, peaches and vanilla essence to a blender. Combine all ingredients in a blender to create a smooth mix

Place grapes, chopped apples and pineapples in an ice-cold bowl. Mix together the mixture. Let the fruit mixture cool in the refrigerator for about 5 minutes. Or, serve it immediately topped with maple syrup.

Salad with Blue and Red Fruits

Ingredients

1/4 cup of sliced prunes

1/4 cup chopped apricots

Blue berries 1/4 cup

1/4 cup of Raspberries

1 tsp. cinnamon powder

1/4 cup of chopped mint leaves

Raw honey 1 tbsp.

2 tbsp. orange juice

Method

Mix all the chopped fruits together in a large bowl. Incorporate the mint leaves, cinnamon powder, and salt. Combine the raw honey with orange juice in a small saucepan. Mix well and add to the salad. Give it a good stir and let cool.

Tapioca Fruit Surprise

Ingredients

1/4 cup cubed cucumber

1/4 cup cubed pineapples

Cubed red apples: 1/4 cup

Ripe fresh mango pulp : 1/2 cup

Sliced bananas 1/4 cup

Prunes : 1/4 cup

1/4 cup cooked tapioca

Grated coconut: 1/4 cup

Method

* Arrange cooked tapioca onto a platter

* Place all the cut fruits, prunes and other ingredients in a bowl.

* Mix the mango pulp with the grated coconut.

Assorted Fruit Mix

Ingredients

Red cherries : 1/4 cup

1/4 cup chopped kiwifruit

1/4 cup pomegranate seed

1/2 cup cubed red apples

Cubed pineapple : 1/4 cup

Cubed Papaya : 1/4 cup

Red cherry syrup - 1 tsp.

Basil leaves : 1/4 Cup

Method

All ingredients should be placed in a large bowl. Add the chopped basil leaves to the bowl. Mix all the ingredients together. Serve at room temperature or chilled.

Vegetable Salad

Quinoa Tomato Mint Salad

Ingredients

Al dente cooked quinoa : 3/4 cup

Chopped cucumber - 1/4 cup

Halved cherry tomatoes - 1/2 cup

Chopped parsley 2 tbsp

1 tbsp chopped mint leaves

Salt : As per taste

For salad dressing

Extra virgin olive Oil - 1/2 Cup

Fresh lemon juice - 2 tbsp

Sweet chili flakes - 1 tsp.

Method

* Mix all the ingredients together in a large bowl.

* Mix lemon juice, chili flakes and olive oil together. Slowly stir in olive oil. Season salad dressing with salt. Add to salad bowl. Mix and serve.

Salad Healthy

Ingredients

Chopped cucumbers: 1/4 cup

Chopped tomatoes 1/4 cup

Boiled chickpeas 1 cup

1/4 cup cubed and boiled potatoes

Finely chopped Parsley: 1/4 cup

Fresh lemon juice 1 tbsp

Salt : 1/2 tbsp.

Method

* Combine all ingredients in a large bowl. Stir well

Creamy Squash Salad

Ingredients

1/2 cup chopped yellow bell Pepper

Yellow cherry tomatoes - 1/2 cup

1/3 cup Sweet corn

Fresh dill : 3 tbsp.

Chopped celery 3 tbsp

Fresh mint leaves : 5-6

Yellow squash - 3 to 4

Salt : As per taste

Method

* Peel and cut the squash.

* Blend all ingredients together in a blender to create a fine mixture

* Add the mixture to the spiralized squash. Serve creamy squash salad chilled (or at room temperature).

Vegan Sweet Potato Avocado Cream Salad

Ingredients

1 cup of baby potatoes

Large ripe avocado:1

Dill:1/3 cup

Chopped celery: 1/3 cup

For dressing

Dijon mustard:1 tbsp.

Lemon juice 1 tsp

Smoked paprika:1/4 tsp.

1/4 teaspoon.

Honey:1 tsp.

Salt :As per taste

Method

Baby potatoes should be cooked to al dente. Cut potatoes into half. Peel the potatoes if needed and place in a large bowl.

*Mash avocado. Blend together the dressing ingredients until you get a nice creamy dressing.

*Add avocado dressing and fresh herbs. Toss gently until potatoes are coated evenly. Refrigerate and serve chilled

Tangy Salad

Ingredients

1 cup sliced red tomatoes

1/4 cup of sliced cucumber

1/4 cup Sliced Radish

Finely chopped Parsley:2 Tbsp

Fresh lemon juice:1 Tbsp

1 Sliced green chilli:

Sugar: 1 pinch

Salt:As per taste

Method

Blend all ingredients together in a blender. Combine all ingredients in a blender.

Breakfast recipes

Quinoa Coconut Milk Poridge

Ingredients

Quinoa:3/4 cup

Shredded coconut:1/2 cup

Coconut milk:1 cup

Bay leaf 1

1/2 tsp.

Grated jaggery 1/4 cup

Method

*Soak quinoa overnight and then boil water to make it soft.

*Pour coconut milk into a saucepan. Add bay leaf, cardamom and cardamom powder. Bring milk back to a boil. Stir in cooked quinoa, grated jaggery. Turn heat down to medium-low, stirring frequently until jaggery has melted. Turn off heat. Serve warm

Quinoa Oatmeal with Toasted Almonds

Ingredients

Quinoa: 1/2 cup

Cooked quick oats:1/2 cup

Soy milk 1 1/2 Cup

Sliced Bananas:1

Toasted almonds - 1 tbsp

Vanilla essence:1 tsp.

Maple syrup:1 Tbsp.

Method

*Soak quinoa in water for at least one night. Let quinoa cool in water for at least an hour.

*Add cooked quinoa, oats, and soymilk to a breakfast dish.

*Add all the ingredients and mix well with a fork.

Scrambled tofu served with fresh vegetables

Ingredients

Olive oil: 1 tbsp

Mashed silken tofu:1 cup

Chopped spinach:1 bunch

1. Medium size of sliced bell pepper

Chopped tomato:1 small size

Finely sliced green Chilies: 1 Tbsp

Salt:As per taste

Method

*Heat olive fat in a skillet. Saute bell peppers and green chilies. Stir in chopped spinach.

Add the chopped tomatoes and season it with salt. Cook for a few more minutes until the spinach is tender. Mix in the mashed tofu. Cook for few minutes more

*Serve scrambled Tofu with fresh vegetables and brown bread.

Super food breakfast

Ingredients

Overnight soaked quinoa:1/2 cup

Soaked raisins:Fistful

Grated jaggery 3/4 cup

1/4 cup grated coconut

Coconut milk:1 cup

Green cardamom Powder: 1/2 tsp.

Method

*Pour 1 cup of water into a medium-sized pan. Heat to boiling. Reduce heat, add quinoa, and cook until it absorbs the water.

Bring coconut milk to a boil in a saucepan Mix in the grated coconut, jaggery, and cooked Quinoa. Cook for a few seconds.

Mix in the soaked raisins and greencardamom powder. Stir. Superfood breakfasts can be served hot or cold depending on how you like it.

Coconut Stuffed Pancakes

Ingredients

Coconut oil 2 tbsp

Overnight soaked rice:1 cup

Grated jaggery - 1 cup

1 1/2 cups grated coconut

Soaked raisins:Fistful

Method

Make pancakes by blending soaked rice, water and flour in a blender.

*In saucepan, heat grated jaggery until it turns sticky. Stir in the grated coconut. Keep stirring to create a sticky mix. Add in the soaked raisins. Mix well, then turn off the heat.

Heat coconut oil in a saucepan. Make pancakes with the rice mixture. Top with the cooked jaggery/coconut mixture. Make pancakes with the leftover batter, and then stuff with the coconut mixture. Serve warm coconut stuffed pancakes

Main Course Lunch/Dinner

Spicy Lentil Vegetable Curry

Ingredients

Olive oil: 1 tbsp

Cumin seeds:1 teaspoon

1 cup cooked lentil

Chopped cabbage:1/4 cup

1 cup of sliced tomatoes

1/4 cup cubed potatoes or carrots

Green peas - 1/4 cup

1/4 cup chopped French beans

Turmeric powder: 1 teaspoon

Red chili powder: 1 teaspoon

Ginger paste:1 tbsp.

Salt:T tbsp.

Method

*Heat the oil in a large skillet. Stir in cumin seeds. Toss all vegetables with the exception of tomatoes. Cook vegetables for few minutes

*Add red chili powder and turmeric powder to the skillet. Then add the tomatoes. Continue cooking on low heat until the tomatoes become tender.

*Add cooked lentils, season with salt, toss in the vegetables and bring to a boil.

* Serve warm lentil vegetable curry with steamed brown potatoes

Mixed Vegetable Rice Soup
Ingredients

Brown rice cooked in 1 cup

Olive oil: 1 TSP

Vegetable broth:2 1/2 cups

Large size tomatoes:1

1/4 cup Peeled and diced potatoes

Broccoli florets 1/4 cup

Peeled and diced carrots: 1/4 cup

Sweet peas - 1/4 cup

Chopped baby cabbage, 1/4 cup

Grated ginger 1 tsp

Lemon grass: 1 bag

Salt:As per taste

Black pepper powder 1 tsp.

Finely chopped Parsley: 1 Tbsp

Method

*Microwave tomatoes until they are soft. Peel the skins off the tomatoes, then mash them in a bowl.

Microwave all the vegetables to tenderize. For 1 minute more, add the mashed tomato and microwave.

*In large soup pot, combine vegetable broth, cooked vegetables. Add cooked rice, grated ginger, and lemongrass. Bring the soup back to boil. Turn off heat and add lemon juice.

*Season soup seasoned with salt and pepper Warm mixed vegetable soup, garnished warm with chopped parsley

Aromatic Vegetable and Rice

Ingredients

Rice:1 Cup

Olive oil:1 1/2 Tablespoon

Green cardamom pods:2

Cinnamon 3 inch

Cloves:4

Peeled and cubed potatoes, carrots, and potatoes: 1/2 cup

1/4 cup shelled peas

1/4 cup chopped French beans

Turmeric powder: 1/2 teaspoon

Sugar: A pinch

Slit green chilies:2

Chopped mint leaves 2 tbsp

Salt :As per taste

Method

*Soak rice in half-hour of water

*Heat olive oils in a pressure cooker at medium heat. Stir in the dry spices. Allow to sit for at least a minute so that the flavors can infuse. Sauté for a minute, adding the green chilies, sugar, herbs, and spices.

*Now add vegetables and turmeric powder. Cook on medium heat for a few minutes. Mix the soaked rice into the vegetables. Cook on medium heat for about 5 minutes, or until the vegetables and rice are cooked well. Stir in 2 cups water. Season with salt.

*Open the pressure cooker's lid and cook until rice is done. Serve aromatic vegetable-rice warm

Mashed Seasoned Kartoffels

Ingredients

Large potatoes:2

Seasoning

1 tsp.

Finely chopped parsley. 1/4 cup

Salt:As per taste

Method

*Boil potatoes till al dente. Peel skins and roughly mash them. Mix the seasoning ingredients with a fork.

Gingery Beet Carrot Sauce

Ingredients

Peeled and cubed beets - 1/2 cup

Peeled and cubed carrots 1/2 cup

Finely grated ginger: 1 teaspoon

Finely chopped Parsley: 1 teaspoon

Bay leaf 1

Vegetable broth:1 1/2 cup

Salt:As per taste

Method

*In a large saucepan pour vegetable broth. Blend in the bay leaves and grated ginger. Bring everything to a boil.

When the broth is boiling, add the chopped veggies and continue cooking. Season with salt, pepper, and turn off heat

Allow the soup time to cool. Blend the soup with a blender until it becomes a fine liquid.

*Bring the soup back to boil in a saucepan. Change the heat. Warm gingerybeet carrot soup garnished with chopped Parsley

Lemony Steamed Vegetables
Ingredients

Broccoli florets - 1/4 cup

Fresh green peas - 1/4 cup

Peeled and chopped carrots: 1/4 cup

1/4 cup Peeled, cubed potatoes

Summer squash:1/4 cup

Fresh lemon leaves

Fresh ground black Pepper: 1 teaspoon

Lemon zest:1 tsp.

Oregano:1/2 tsp.

Salt:As per taste

Method

*Wash all vegetables well under running water.

*To steam the vegetables, place them in a steamer. The lemon leaves can be shredded and tossed into the steamer. Steam cook the vegetables to al dente

*Place the steam vegetables in a bowl. Sprinkle with pepper powder and lemon zest. Season the dish with salt, salt, and/oregano. Combine all ingredients and toss. Serve warm with lemony steamed vegetables

Tofu and Vegetables with Rice Noodles

Ingredients

Al dente cooked rice noodles:1/2 cup

Olive oil: 1 1/2 Tablespoon

Medium-sized bell pepper

Medium size carrot:1

Fresh bean sprouts:1/2 cup

Grated ginger 1 tsp

Chopped green chilies:1 teaspoon

Tofu:1 pc

Soy sauce:3 tbsp.

Fresh lemon juice: 2 Tbsp

Brown sugar: 1 Tbsp

Salt:Salt according to your taste

Method

*Press tofu gently between two paper towels to drain excess liquid. Cut tofu in 1 inch cubes

*Cut the carrots into thin strips. Cut bell pepper into thin strips

*In small bowl combine soy sauce with sugar and lime juice

*In large skillet heat oil. Add grated ginger, green chilies and garlic. Stir in vegetables, and cook for a few more minutes. Season with salt if necessary. Add the cubed Tofu and 3/4th cup of the mixed sauces to the pan. Continue stirring-frying until vegetables are almost cooked.

*Add the cooked noodles to the pan and continue stirring-frying for about 5 minutes. Transfer to a platter, add the remaining sauce and then serve.

Beet and Carrot Pasta Noodles with Spicy Vegetables

Ingredients

1.25 cups of spiralized, peelable carrots and beets

1/2 cup of stewed dark red kidney bean soup

Baby potatoes:1/4 cup

Sweet peas - 1/4 cup

1/4 cup chopped green bell pepper

Chopped cabbage:1/4 cup

Chop tomatoes with juice: 1 1/2 cup

Olive oil 1 1/2 tbsp.

Seasoning: 1 TSP

Cumin seeds:1 teaspoon

Red chili powder:1 teaspoon

Cumin powder: 1 teaspoon

Turmeric powder: 1/2 teaspoon

Salt:As per taste

Method

*Heat olive-oil in a large saucepan. Saute spiralized carrots & beets.

*Heat olive oils in a pressure cooker. Then crackle cumin seed. Chop tomatoes and all seasoning ingredients. Season with salt, and heat on medium heat to melt the oil.

*Add the vegetables to the pressure cooker. Cook for a few more minutes. Cover the pressure cooker with a lid and let it cook for several minutes, or until the vegetables are tender. Turn off the pressure cooker and place the cooked beans inside. Continue cooking for a few minutes.

*In a platter, arrange the sauteed carrots. Serve the cooked vegetables over the pasta. Serve beets and carrots noodles warm with spicy vegetables

Raw Mango Vegetable Mixed

Ingredients

Medium size plantain:1

Medium potato:1

Medium sweet potato:1

Small size ash gourds:1

Medium raw mango 1

Broccoli florets 1/2 cup

Slit green chilies:2

Chopped celery stalk 1/4 cup

Curry leaves: 1/4 cup

Turmeric powder: 1 teaspoon

Fresh pounded pepper -1/2 tsp.

Salt:As per taste

Method

*Peel and wash plantain and sweet potato. Cut into 2 inch-long pieces.

*To remove bitterness from the plantain, mix salt, turmeric powder, and a small amount of water.

Bring the water to boil in large saucepan. Stir in all the vegetables and season with salt, turmeric powder, celery stalk, green chilies, and salt.

*Add the chopped raw mango slices, black pepper powder and curry leaves to the vegetables. Continue to boil over medium heat, stirring occasionally, until vegetables are al dente. Transfer the vegetables to a platter. Serve warm

Hot and Sweet Burritos

Ingredients

1 Green baby cabbage

Purple baby cabbage

Red carrot:1

Sweet pepper:1

Peeled zucchini:1

Chopped celery: 1/4 cup

Peeled and diced mangoes:1/2 cup

For dressing

Chili Flakes:1 tsp.

Orange Juice:2 Tbsp.

Black salt:1 tsp.

Method

*In a food processer, blend the burrito ingredients until they form a fine texture. Mix the ingredients in a bowl.

In a small bowl, whisk together all the dressing ingredients. Mix it well and then pour the mixture over. Mix in the diced mangoes. Mix all ingredients using a fork. Enjoy hot and sweet burritos by placing them in the outer half of the cabbage leaves.

Protein Punch

Ingredients

Split green gram:1/2 cup

Sunflower oil:1 Tbsp.

Turmeric powder:1 teaspoon

Salt:As per taste

Method

*Soak spit-green gram for at least a couple of hours. Once the spit green has become tender, pressure cook it with 1 cup water and turmeric powder. Make sure to check the consistency. If needed, you can add more hotwater.

*Put olive oil in the pan. Add cumin seeds. Mix tempering with the cooked greengram.

Carrot Beetroot Fry w/ Shredded Coconut

Ingredients

Coconut oil: 1 Tbsp.

Cumin seeds:1 teaspoon

Red chili:1

Curry leaves:6-8

Turmeric powder:1 teaspoon

Green peas - 1/4 cup

Half a cup of sliced carrots

1 cup chopped beetroots

1/4 cup of shredded coconut

Method

*Heat coconut butter in a large saucepan. Add cumin seeds. Curry leaves. Stir-fry the vegetables with cumin seeds, curry leaves, and broken red chili until well coated.

*Incorporate shredded coconut, and saute for 1 minute

Cinnamon Vegetable Soup

Ingredients

Olive oil

Bay leaves:2

Whole black pepper:5-6

2" Cinnamon bark:1

Grated ginger 1 tsp

Chopped celery stalk - 1 tbsp

One cup of chopped mixed vegetables

Chopped leafy vegetable:1/2 cup

Vegetable stock:2 cup

Brown sugar: 1/2 tsp.

Cinnamon powder: 1/2 teaspoon

Salt:as per taste

Method

In a wok heat the olive oil. Stir in bay leaves and whole black pepper. Add cinnamon for a light brown color. Saute ginger and celery stalk. Combine all vegetables and saute for about one minute.

*Now, add the dry spice and continue to sautee the vegetables. Mix vegetable stock with sugar. Season the mixture with cinnamon powder, salt, and sugar. Bring to boil. Turn down heat. Cook the vegetables until al dente. Turn off heat. Arrange and serve warm.

Red Pasta with Tofu & Vegetables
Ingredients

Al dente boiled penne pasta:1 cup

Olive oil: 1 Tbsp.

Grated ginger 1 tsp

Chopped red bell peppers:1/2 cup

Shredded Cabbage 1/2 Cup

Cubed Tofu: 1/2 cup

Cherry tomatoes halved: 1/2 cup

Salt:as per taste

Dry spices

Red paprika Flour: 1 tsp.

Oregano:1 tsp.

Fresh pepper powder: 1 teaspoon

Method

*Heat olive oil in the wok. Once it is hot, add grated ginger. Sauté all the vegetables for a few moments. Sprinkle with dry spices, and give it a toss. Season with salt, pepper, and then add sliced tomatoes. Stir fry for few minutes till tomatoes soften

*Add the boiled pasta to the mixture and toss. Transfer to a platter.

Pasta in rich tomato gravy

Ingredients

Al dente boiled pasta:1 cup

Olive oil 2 tbsp

1

medium size ripe sweet tomatoes:4

Grated ginger 1 tsp

Chopped green chilies: 1 tsp.

Chopped red bell peppers:1/2 cup

Chopped carrots:1/2 cup

1/2 cup cubed tofu

Chopped cilantro:1 TSP

Salt:as per taste

Dry spices

Oregano:1 tsp.

Basil:1 tsp.

Chili flakes:1 tsp.

1 teaspoon pepper powder

Method

*Heat olive oil using a pressure cooker. Saute the tomatoes and capsicums in olive oil for about a minute. Turn the heat to medium and close the pressure cooker. Allow the mixture to cool down to room temperature. Then, use a mixer to combine all the ingredients.

*Heat olive oil on a pan. Saute the ginger and green chilies. Stir-fry the chopped vegetables and tofu. Mix all the ingredients well.

*Now, add the cooked pasta. Season it with dry spices and salt. Mix together all ingredients. Serve with chopped cilantro.

Chili Tofu Noodles

Ingredients

Al dente boiled noodles:1 cup

Olive oil: 1 Tbsp.

Grated ginger 1 tsp

3

Cubed Tofu: 1/2 cup

1/2 cup chopped green bell pepper and red bell peper

Chopped Chinese cabbage:1/4 cup

1/4 teaspoon pepper powder

Salt:as per taste

For sauce

Tomato sauce:1 tsp.

Red chili sauce:1 tsp.

Soy sauce:1 tsp.

Lemon juice 1 tsp

Method

*Heat olive ole in a wok. Saute the ginger and green chillies. Toss with vegetables and tofu

*In a large bowl, combine all sauce ingredients. Season the vegetables well with salt and pepper. Stir in the boiled noodles. Stir fry for a few more minutes before serving.

Red Kidney Beans Curry

Ingredients

Olive oil:1 tbsp

Peanut butter: 1 Tbsp

Kidney beans: 1 cup

Grated ginger 1 tbsp

One cup of chopped tomatoes with juice

Garam masala powder:1/2 tsp.

Salt:as per taste

Dry spices

Cinnamon stick, 3 inch

Use cardamom to make:3

Cloves:4

Spice powder

Turmeric powder:1 teaspoon

Red chili powder:1 teaspoon

1 tsp. coriander and cumin powder

Method

*Soak 1-cup kidney beans in 2 cups of water for at least overnight. Pressure cook the soaked kidneys until tender with enough water and 1 tablespoon peanut butter.

*Heat the olive oil in an ovenproof pan. Once it has melted, add all of the dry spices. Allow them to brown. Grate the ginger and stir in chopped tomatoes. Season with dry spices. Toss in the chopped tomatoes and olive oil.

*Add cooked beans, season with salt, and continue cooking for a few minutes. Bring 1 cup water to a boil. Add a pinch Garam Masala and stir. Turn off heat and let cool down before serving.

Asparagus, Red Quinoa Salad

Ingredients

Mustard oil 1 tbsp

Nigella seeds:1/2 tsp.

Slit green chili:1-2

Cooked red quinoa:1 cup

Sliced asparagus:1 Cup

1/2 cup sliced radish

Salt:as per taste

Method

*Heat mustard oil in pan. Add the nigellas seeds and let them splutter. Season the dish with salt and add all the vegetables. Stir-fry all the ingredients until they are cooked. Let cool for a couple of minutes before serving.

Hot and Sweet Quinoa Bowl

Ingredients

Olive oil: 1 Tbsp.

Half a cup of boiled Quinoa

1/4 cup of boiled black beans

Tomato pulp:1 cup

2 Sliced green chilies

Paprika:1 tsp.

Sweet corn kernels:1/4 cup

1/2 tsp.

Kosher Salt: A taste

Chopped cilantro:1 Tbsp

Method

Heat the olive oil in an ovenproof pan. Add the tomato pulp along with the slit chilies and paprika. Allow to simmer for five minutes. Then add the boiled black beans and quinoa. Adjust the water to your liking. Season with salt & pepper.

*Bring the mixture to a boil. Then add the sweet corn kernels. Cook the corn till softened. Stir in chopped cilantro. Serve warm.

Coconut Gravy and Plantain with Tofu
Ingredients

Coconut oil: 1 Tbsp.

Cumin seeds: 1 teaspoon

1/2 cup chopped plantain

Tofu cubed: 1/2 cup

Cooked quinoa:1/4 cup

3/4 cup of chopped cherry tomatoes

Kosher Salt: Per taste

Brown sugar: Larger pinch

Curry paste

Cumin seeds:1 teaspoon

Green chilies:2

Grated coconut 1 tbsp

Turmeric:1/2 tsp.

Method

*Mix curry paste ingredients in a small amount of water to make a smooth paste

*Heat coconut oils in a large saucepan. Add cumin seeds. Tofu and curry paste can be sautéed. Stir-fry the cherry tomatoes for a few moments before adding them to the pan. Season with salt, and cook the tomatoes until softened.

*Add cooked quinoa and 1/2 cup water to bring to boil. Remove from heat and stir in the quinoa.

Beet and Carrot Noodles With Mashed Black Bean

Ingredients

Medium size carrots:2-3

Beets medium in size:1

Olive oil: 1 tbsp

Grated ginger 1 tsp

Chopped sweet tomatoes:1 cup

1/2 cup of mashed or cooked black bean

Chopped cilantro:1 tablespoon

Kosher Salt: Per taste

Brown sugar: Larger pinch

Seasoning

Oregano:1/2 tsp.

Black pepper powder 1/2 tsp.

Dry basil: 1/2 tsp.

Method

*Peel and spiralize carrots. Place the olive oil in a large pot and heat it. Stir fry the carrots and beets.

*Heat olive oils in the same pan. Once it is hot, add chopped tomatoes and bell pepper. Add chopped tomatoes, bell pepper and salt. Season with salt, and let cook until tomatoes are tender. Mash the black bean in a small bowl and add it to the tomatoes.

*Fry the mixture for about 5 minutes. Mix in 1/2 cup water. Bring to a boil. The mixture should be poured over the stir-fried carrots, beets, and potatoes. Serve with chopped cilantro

Sweet and Sour Steamed Vegetables Bowl
Ingredients

Mixed vegetables of your choosing: 1 1/2 cups

Salt:as per taste

Dressing:

Olive oil: 1/2 cup

Lemon juice: 2 tbsp

Orange juice: 1 Tbsp

Dry basil 1 tsp

Sweet paprika 1 tsp.

Method

*Steam cook vegetables

For dressing, whisk together all the ingredients. Add olive oil drop-by. Pour dressing over steamed vegetables. Season with salt. Stir well before serving

Tempered Quinoa with Vegetables

Ingredients

Cooked quinoa:1 cup

Coconut oil 2 tbsp

Asafoetida:1 pinch

Grated ginger 1 tsp

Chopped carrots - 1/4 cup

1/4 cup chopped bell pepper

Green peas - 1/4 cup

Half a cup of chopped tomatoes with juice

Turmeric powder: 1/2 teaspoon

Red chili powder:1/2 tsp.

Cumin powder: 1 teaspoon

Chopped cilantro:

Salt:as per taste

For tempering

Curry leaves 5-6

Mustard seeds 1/4 tsp

Cumin:1/2 tsp.

www.ingramcontent.com/pod-product-compliance
Lightning Source LLC
Chambersburg PA
CBHW060326030426
42336CB00011B/1220